NEVER ACCEPT
—— YOUR ——
NEW NORMAL

THE STORY OF USING NEUROSCIENCE
—— TO ——
TURN TRAUMA INTRO TRIUMPH

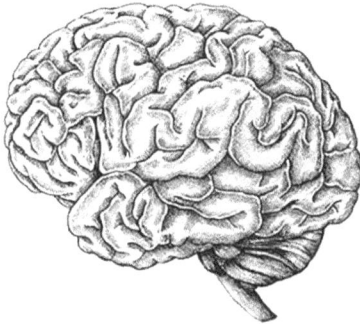

MICHAEL LONGYEAR DC, DACNB, CCSP

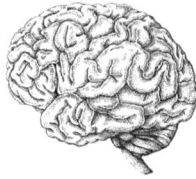

This book is dedicated to…

Everyone that has ever been told, "this is as good as you get" or "you can't get any better" and defied the odds, pushed through and persevered.

DEDICATION

In the middle of difficulty lies opportunity.
—Albert Einstein

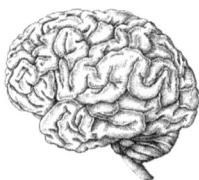

CONTENTS

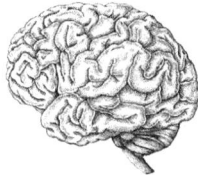

ACKNOWLEDGMENTS

This was the hardest part of this book to write. There have been so many people in my life that have molded, shaped and guided me to this point in my life, and to all of them I am grateful. If I were to write the personal thank that each of you deserves, it would be longer than this book. So, for this book I am going to keep my thank you's to those specific to the journey through my injury and in teaching me how to use that to be better for my patients.

Meaghan, my loving wife. I don't really even know where to begin. Your belief in me always surpassed my belief in myself and that is what has kept me going. You sacrificed to get us through school the first time and to help me realize this book was possible and to push through getting it done. As this book took shape, you dealt with all the mood swings that came as a result of opening up the wounds to heal from them. None of who I am today is possible without you. We have come a long way together and have so much further to go. With you by my side I feel like we can accomplish anything. I LOVE YOU!

Mom, you never let me quit, anything. You have always instilled a work ethic in Chris and I that has always had us striving to finish and be the best we can be. Watching you do things constantly, even though you were told you couldn't, has always been a source of inspiration and strength. You always fight and move forward no matter what you are faced with. You were the first and biggest example of never accepting your new normal, you go get what you want.

Dad, you have been there for me to vent to and get things off my chest. You never judge or look down on me for anything. Even at my lowest points in life you have always known what to say to lift me up and always known when to say it too. Thank you for always believing in me, even when I have not believed in myself.

Chris, even as a younger brother I always looked to you for strength, sometimes literally. You always motivated me to be a better person and a better big brother by the example you set. A big part of my motivation to play football again and to push myself was to get to play one year with you on the team.

Dr. Michael J. Brown, thank you for getting me back on track and getting me to chiropractic school so I could begin to realize my purpose again. Without your nudge, I would have never started the journey.

Dr. Fritz Boehm, thank you for the adjustment that gave me back my sensation and would eventually help me realize my purpose and passion.

Dr. Michael Hall, thank you for mentoring, guiding and imparting your wisdom to me. Trying to figure out how your brain could see ten steps ahead all the time kept me striving to be better and learn more. I realize now how far ahead of the curve your teaching put all of us students that had the opportunity to learn from you. Ultimately, thank you for showing me the lens I needed to use to view the patient.

Dr. Len Wisneski, thank you for being a friend, a mentor and for really teaching me how to handle the gifts that were given to me by others. You showed me how to take my knowledge and compassion and how to use it with others but most importantly not to burn myself out and give all my energy while doing it. And for getting me to realize my gifts of bringing things together to think outside the box. You showed me the lens with which I view myself with the patient.

Dr. Gilles LaMarche, your mentoring on professionalism and how to approach each day has changed me as a person, as a doctor and made me grow in ways I never thought I would or could grow. I always strive to come from a place of service and love because that is the example that you have set and that you personify every day and in everything you do.

Jon Vestal, you have always been a sound board for me and always told me the truth. Especially when I didn't want to hear it. You always let me rant and blow off steam without challenging me at the wrong time.

Luke Skiera, you stood by me in my return and made getting back to my life after the trauma seem normal. You never let me feel broken as I healed and always made sure I was included in things and got into trouble with me to keep my mind off things. The saying or joke that always comes to mind from those times is the one about how to tell a good friend from a best friend. A good friend will come bail you out of jail when you get into trouble, but a best friend is sitting in the cell next to you.

NEVER ACCEPT YOUR NEW NORMAL

**The Neuroscience Behind Turning
Trauma into Triumph**

A Challenge for You

As you start reading this book, I want you to think about those times people told you to "just give up" or "that might be too hard" or, my personal favorite, "this is as good as you're going to get." Those words are limitations. They are OPINIONS, not the ultimate truth.

If you have overcome a limitation in health or in any other aspect of your life, I want you to post what you were told and how you proved them wrong with the hashtag **#NeverAcceptYourNewNormal**, and tag this Facebook Account: **Facebook.com/neveracceptyournewnormal**. I want to show our collective stories to people who are taking those limitations to heart, to give them hope.

This book is about my personal journey and the journeys of other patients of mine who chose not to accept their new normal. Because we did so, we get to enjoy a happier, more fulfilled life enjoying things we were told we may never get to do again.

This book uses actual patient case studies to help describe some complex neurological conditions. The names and likeness of these patients have been changed to protect patient anonymity in accordance with HIPAA guidelines.

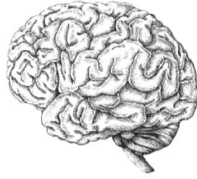

CHAPTER ONE

THE BEGINNING OF MY STORY

Suddenly my mind lunged to alertness. At first, my living room looked a little blurry and fuzzy as I shook off the grogginess from last night's pain meds and muscle relaxers. I felt the couch's synthetic polyester fabric and saw the loud wallpaper and popcorn ceiling, customary for an old home still clinging to its Victorian roots. I smelled the cold and felt the chill of November in northern Michigan. I relaxed for a moment, comfortable in my surroundings.

My mouth was dry and the feeling of cotton on my tongue made me thirsty. I attempted to stand up from the couch, but I was met with resistance and confusion. For some reason, my legs didn't want to swing off the couch. For a split second I thought I was dreaming, or that my legs were asleep. That belief was shattered by the realization that I couldn't even *feel* my legs when I touched them. Before I fully realized I was doing it, I released a scream of confusion and fear. My brain figured out that my body wasn't working.

The first person I saw coming down the stairs was my mother with a look of fright on her face. She heard the scream and came to see what the hell was going on. The next twenty minutes are a blur in my memory. Some of the neighbors showed up to see if everything was alright, and then the paramedics came. My mind was still trying to wrap itself around what was going on, still hoping this was all a dream. When they tried to pick me up from the couch and put weight on my legs, the movement of straightening my body was met with excruciating spasms in my stomach and abdomen, causing me to fall back to the couch in agony. Before I knew it, I was being loaded onto a stretcher and then wheeled out to the ambulance. The crisp morning air hit my face as we exited the house. At that point, I became completely sure that I wasn't dreaming.

My mind swirled at a dizzying pace during the short trip to the hospital. In this small town, nothing was too far away. We arrived at the hospital, and the waiting and testing began. I was loaded into a CT scan machine, then an MRI. Nurses ran in and out of my room, coming to check on me. The doctors came to check my chart and go over test results with my mom. Each test yielded no answers, just more confusion for the doctors. For eight hours I sat, hoping and praying that my legs would wake up and start to move again. I begged the universe to let me get up and walk out of the hospital. I hoped that the doctors would give me some answers soon.

No answers came.

As I was sitting there, my thoughts drifted back to the night before. I was at my high school, decorating the halls for homecoming week. Had something last night triggered this? My buddy Luke and I had snuck in a few sips of liquor out of his dad's cabinet before heading up to the school. It seemed pretty innocent at the time, but had that liquor caused such a reaction?

My blood went cold. Was it an injury from the football game two days ago? I couldn't remember getting hit any harder than usual…

Even after an eternity, the doctors couldn't figure out what was going on. They loaded me up in an ambulance for an hour-long drive to another hospital. This hospital was in a bigger city with more doctors who specialize in conditions like mine. They also had, the doctors said, "groundbreaking, specialized technology" that their hospital didn't.

I shouldn't have been surprised that this hospital couldn't come to a conclusion. After all, I was here just yesterday, and they missed this upcoming problem. The night before, while I was at the high school putting up decorations, I had a bit of tightness in my chest. It got so bad that I started to have trouble breathing, so I had my buddy Luke drive me home to let my mom know what was going on (this was before cell phones). By the time I got home after the roughly one-mile trip, breathing was so difficult we decided to go to the emergency room.

Upon arriving, they asked the normal questions, then set me aside in the waiting room. When we finally got called back, they ordered the standard tests for a kid complaining of tightness in the chest who had just played football a day earlier. They ran an X-ray, poked me with a few reflex hammers, and sent me home with a prescription for a muscle relaxer and a pain med. Their diagnosis was of a pulled muscle and an out-of-place rib. Not very thorough, but I wasn't questioning them (yet). After all, they were the experts, and I was only fifteen years old—who was I to argue?

By the time we got home, I was really struggling to make it up the front stairs. I had to lean on my mom and stepdad to climb just six steps. Something wasn't right. As soon as we got in the house, we called the hospital and told them about this new symptom. They immediately dismissed it as the effects of the medication on my body. I slowly made my way to the couch, pretty fatigued from summiting the stairs. I lay down to watch TV and drifted to sleep pretty quickly. Not twenty-four hours later, I was on my way to Traverse City in an ambulance, unable to feel the lower half of my body and unsure what my future would hold. I was scared for my life.

When we arrived, they unloaded my broken body from the ambulance and began to wheel me into the hospital on the stretcher. A neurologist, Dr. Beard, met us before they even got me through the doors. He is gray-haired with a scraggly beard, and he is carrying a safety pin and a Magic Marker. This was, apparently, the "groundbreaking, specialized technology" they sent me up there for. He stopped the stretcher and pulled the neck of my hospital gown down just below my chest. He poked me in the shoulder with his safety pin and asked me if it felt sharp.

I replied, "Yes."

He then said, "Tell me when it doesn't feel sharp anymore," and proceeded to continuously poke my chest with his pin.

When he reached a level about even with my nipples, I suddenly could no longer feel the sharp stab of the pin. It felt like he had stopped using the pin and was now poking me gently with his finger. I look down to see if he was trying to trick me, only to find the pin still in his hand, poking me in the chest. I told him that it was no longer sharp.

He grabbed his black Magic Marker and drew a line at that point on my chest, looked at the person next to him, and said, "He has a lesion in his T-spine."

A lesion in my *what*? I had no idea what he had just said, but in the thirty short seconds that I had known this doctor he had already told me more about what was going on than I had heard in eight hours at the other hospital.

The whole time I was in the hospital, my thoughts just kept repeating: *I was only decorating for homecoming; how could this happen? There has to be something else that landed me here. Is it possible it was football? Could it have been a bad tackle from the game two days ago?*

The rest of my time in the second hospital was another blur. I remember hearing bits and pieces that either did not make sense or scared me so much I tried to block them out. At fifteen years old I didn't know a whole lot, but I did understand whispered phrases like "possible MS" and "wheelchair bound." It was pretty devastating to hear those things—and pretty shocking too, especially when, less than seventy-two hours ago, I had been on the gridiron.

At that point it seemed like so long ago that I was normal and able to walk. It's funny how time works during an event like this. During some portions time seems to fly by, but at other points time seems to stand still and take an eternity to pass as you feel like your life is coming to end.

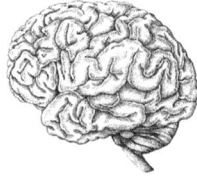

CHAPTER TWO

MY REASON FOR WRITING THIS BOOK

Sometimes, especially when we are in the thick of a situation, it can be hard to understand that things are often not done *to* us by the universe, but *for* us. This story is not about the negatives of what I went through on this journey but rather about how it shaped my outlook on life, health and well-being, and especially health care. It became a driving force for me to learn everything I could about what makes us tick, to better understand myself and what I went through. My injury was, and is, the hardest thing that I have ever gone through—but it is also the thing that most shaped me into who I am today.

My story is, even twenty-five years later, still hard to talk about. I didn't sit down one day and decide to tell my story in this book—rather, I kept this story inside for so long that it clawed its way out when I least expected it.

For a long time, I kept this story in and didn't share it. At one point I even destroyed all the pictures my parents had of me in the hospital. I guess for a while I thought that if I kept it in and ignored it, I wouldn't have to deal with having been broken—or still being broken. At that point I never realized how much my story could be my fuel, passion, and connection to this life.

I kept this story in until one night in 2015, twenty years after the event. I awoke in the middle of the night with memories of my time in the hospital flooding back to me. Quickly after they started, I began to sob uncontrollably. It lasted for what seemed like hours, so I began to write some of them down in the notes section of my phone just to see if trying to activate my thinking brain would quiet my limbic, emotional brain.

If we don't deal with things, they have a way of *making* us deal with them. Sometimes by the time we stop to listen, it can be too late. Our traumas can lay just below the surface and affect our lives in ways we don't realize. They can cause us to be hyper-vigilant or live in fear. This fear will then activate certain networks in our brains—including the limbic system—that keep us from enjoying life, and also decrease our memory, concentration, focus, capacity to love and be social, and especially our ability to control our immune responses to fight off sickness and keep things like cancer at bay.

Those same networks of the brain are also responsible for keeping our autonomic nervous system in check—the whole fight-or-flight versus rest-and-digest part of our nervous system. If we cannot regulate that, we end up with depression, anxiety, and other mental health disorders.

Writing about and finally facing my trauma worked to heal those parts of my brain. As I wrote, I began to cognitively think about the story and what was happening at that time. I was able to hold it back a little. However, memories would still come back in intense flashes for a few nights, each time waking me out of dead sleep to be at the mercy of undealt with emotions.

This book is my therapy. Twenty years past due time, but better late than never, right? Even after writing all my memory flashes down, it never occurred to me to put them together as a book to help others. Then, my mom happened to write a book about how her journey with a dog she adopted helped her through some hard times in her life. That made me put it together that I could use my story to help others.

It's amazing how events can affect us in such different ways depending on perspective. I have always pulled a great deal of strength from my injury and the events I went through. I have always said that I would not wish it on my worst enemy, but I would also never take it back. Our darkest times and most challenging trials are meant to teach us about ourselves. My darkest time has made me who I am.

If something seems insurmountable or difficult, I always draw on the fact that I relearned to walk. I've made it back from having a serious debate with myself about how and why I should end my life. But as much as I've drawn on that experience for strength, it's amazing how much it still weighs me down. Writing this book was an attempt to release the parts of these events that pulled at me so I could move forward with the positive experiences that can be taken out of my journey.

Whatever your religion or focus is, the soul is meant to bear scars. In these scars, we discover who we are and what our purpose is. The ability to draw the positive from these experiences pushes us to a better state as human beings and hopefully allows us to see a purpose for our struggle. This ability also gives us the opportunity to help others when they go through their trials.

Through this book, I hope to share my strength and wisdom so you, too, are able to learn that health and life are active processes, and that a diagnosis is not a death sentence but an opportunity to grow and evolve.

When all you're doing is surviving, you can't dream, and you can't thrive. We want to give hope so people can dream again because out of those dreams can come a change in mind-set, which can then become healing.

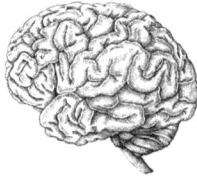

— CHAPTER THREE —

THE ARRIVAL

When I arrived at the second hospital, I was placed on the pediatric floor. I was fifteen, so it makes sense, but I remember being offended by it. As all teens do, I saw myself as an adult, not a child.

Everything was happening very fast. I was pulled into my room, and the curtain was drawn around the bed behind mine in the back of the room. I could hear another family talking behind it as my family got my things situated. I was in and out of the room the first few hours, running from test to test and seeing an endless flow of nurses and doctors. It was all so exhausting. I think I passed out in between different people because my body and brain just couldn't keep up with it.

I do vividly remember waking up for one of the hospital staff and seeing a "get well" balloon above my bed. I was confused as to who would have gotten this for me so soon. After the nurse left, my mom informed me that the boy in the bed next to me was allowed to go home and had told my mom that, since he was allowed to go home, I probably needed it more than he did now.

A confusing feeling came over me. It was the first nice thing that had been done for me that day, but it left me with a pit in my stomach. Was I that bad that even a child knew I was broken and doomed?

The testing was all pretty much a blur, but there is only one test I remember pretty intensely. Knowing what I know now, I can't seem to find a reason for them to have given me this test, unless they were really grasping at straws.

I was face down on a cold metallic table I could feel through my gown. It was so cold on my cheek that it almost hurt. I remember them telling me that I would feel a pressure in the bottom of my spine and that I might feel some pain in the spinal column.

Now this part, I don't know if it is true or if it was just a hallucination from the hospital and drugs, but I still have nightmares about this. I felt the needle running up from the bottom of my spine, and I heard a cracking or crunching in my neck, like the metallic sound of a car crushing, or that sound you hear as you crack open a crab shell in search of meat. This sound is still etched in my mind, as is the searing heat in my neck that came after it. Then the table started to move me around in different directions, almost like one of those immersive 3D roller-coaster rides, but smoother and slower. It was slowly moving left and right, head down and head up, then in different combinations of the movements. It was a tilt table test. I don't know if they were monitoring pressure, or moving a dye around, or what, but whatever it was it felt really creepy.

The recurring dream of this experience feels so real but doesn't make sense or fit into any of what I would now expect a doctor to test for. There was a lot of testing but not a lot of explanation, at least to me. I am sure that they were keeping my mom and dad up to date on the testing, but I was kind of left in the dark without them there to comfort me.

After what seemed like a million tests, Dr. Beard—the man who had poked me with the safety pin—finally walked in to discuss his thoughts with us. He came to the foot of my bed with my chart in his hands. His beady little eyes peered out from behind his glasses, his scraggly gray hair and scraggly gray beard finishing off the look. He definitely looked the part of a nerdy neurologist, and I had endless admiration for him. I was still in awe that he understood what was going on with me using nothing more than a safety pin and black Magic Marker, and I was so excited to hear what he had to say, sure that he'd only bring good news.

He quickly looked up from the chart and said, very coldly, "You have had a spinal infarct or spinal stroke at C7-T1 in your spine. You will never walk again." This was that lesion in my T-spine that he was referring to in our first meeting.

He then looked down, set the chart on the end of the bed, and left the room. My mom quickly followed him, and I could hear mumbles coming from the hallway.

The next thoughts were on how I might be able to end my own life. I was thinking that I could probably get someone to help me, like bring me a gun or something.

The only other gripping thought in my mind was a repeating mantra: *I can't live like this. I can't burden my family like this. I can't live in a wheelchair. I **can't** live like this.*

The Play

The coaches, at the doctors' request, gave my mom the tape to bring to the hospital so the doctors could watch it with me, looking for what might have caused this condition. The doctors were as stumped as I was as to what could have caused this. The only thing that made any sense to them was that it had to have been from the game.

I've watched the tape of my last football game before my injury over and over again, trying to see what may have caused all of this. To this day the images of the game are burned into my memory. I can see that play over and over again, but nothing on the tape or in my memory of the game seemed like it should result in the helpless and pathetic condition my broken body was in. I mean I was hit hard, but I finished the game walking. The only explanation, to them, was a delayed onset inflammatory process from the game that eventually choked off my spinal cord.

The play that my doctors thought could have caused my condition was what we called a "51/61 ends five and out, pass." I was number 84, and on the tape, I was lined up on the right side, one foot away from the right tackle's foot. I played tight end in a wing formation offense—I was the last guy on the line. There is a wing or H-back lined up just behind me and to the outside. On this particular play, my job was to chip the defensive end and release from the line, run up field five yards, make a hard 90 degree cut, and run to the sideline. The ball should be on the way when I stick my foot, and in the air, as I make my turn.

The timing was perfect. As I turned, the ball was on its way. The line of the ball was right, too. It led me into the route; I kept my stride and reached out for the ball that was delivered just over my left shoulder. Just as my hands gripped the ball, my motion was stopped by the defensive back, making his way back in from the sideline on a crackback. His hit was so jarring that I don't remember feeling it. The linebacker hit me in the front shoulder as he trailed me into the route.

They had hit me on opposite shoulders and twisted me to the ground. The three of us went to the ground in a twisted heap. I remember getting up sore from the hit, but it didn't make sense that that one tackle could have caused all this. I didn't even miss a play as a result of the hit. Yeah, it hurt, but not much more than any other hard hit in football. I had been hit harder. But as I watched the play over and over again in the hospital, the understanding that my dreams of any future in athletics would now be unattainable was made obvious.

That instant on the tape, one that had seemed so insignificant, completely changed my life. It had turned me into a crippled mess. At fifteen years old, every hope and dream I had ever had of being a football player was crushed.

The self-pity was pretty strong around that video. Most of my memories of that tape are distorted by my tears. I would watch my future plans slip away, stop, rewind, and watch them slip away again. Looking back, it was pretty pathetic, but I think this process was necessary. I had to allow myself to wallow in that moment of grief for at least a little while.

One of the days that I was there in my hospital bed, painfully re-watching the play, one of the nurses brought me something else to watch. It was *The Dennis Byrd Story*. It had come out in February of that year, 1994.

Byrd was a New York Jets football player who suffered a neck injury in a game against the Kansas City Chiefs on November 29, 1992. The neck injury was so bad it left him paralyzed. The nurse brought in the tape of Byrd's injury and it, like mine, looked pretty benign. He was rushing the quarterback, Dave Krieg, and collided with his teammate, Scott Mersereau, as Krieg stepped up to avoid the sack. Byrd ducked his head out of instinct at the last second before hitting Mersereau in the chest with the top of his head.

The collision broke his fifth cervical vertebrae and damaged the spinal cord leaving him paralyzed. But his story didn't stop there. It continued on. They told him—just like they told me—that he may never walk again, but he did. He was able to rehab and work hard and regained the use of his legs. Byrd returned to the Meadowlands for the Jets' home opener on September 5, 1993, walking to midfield as an honorary captain for the coin toss. During the halftime ceremony, Steve Gutman, the president of the Jets, presented him with a trophy for the Most Inspirational Player Award, which would thereafter be called the Dennis Byrd Award.

This video couldn't have come at a better time. This guy took his injury and used it as fuel to push himself. He got out of his chair and eventually even walked on the field again. It was a huge inspiration. I had proof that I could get out of the chair, even if they said it wasn't possible.

To Walk or Not to Walk, That is the Question

What is the point? I thought as they wheeled my fairly lifeless body through the catacombs of the hospital. I was on my way to my first day in physical therapy, having just been told a few days earlier that I would never walk again. When I first got there, the physical therapy director came over to talk with me. He told me that his orders were to teach me how to use my wheelchair (even now, as I type those words, tears well up in my eyes) since this would be my method of transportation for the foreseeable future. Since I wouldn't be able to walk again, I needed to know how to do everything there is to do with a wheelchair.

As a fifteen-year-old, this seemed completely stupid. *What is there to teach me?* Sitting down, grabbing the wheels, and push-ing—seemed pretty self-explanatory to me. All I kept asking was if we were going to work on getting me to walk. And all they kept saying was "No."

Since my case was pretty cut and dry, they stuck me with an intern, Natalie, who was there getting her credits for classes. I say "stuck" because that is how I felt when they explained this to me, but little did I know that she would be the best person for me. She explained to me that she would be teaching me how to use my chair, but also the ins and outs of safety—like what to do if I fell out of the chair, and how to not tip backward.

Tip backward? That was about the only interesting thing to fifteen-year-old me. Thinking about popping wheelies was the only thing that picked up my mood for a second. Besides wheelies, there was nothing appealing about a wheelchair to a kid who had been on the football field catching touchdown passes a week ago.

I am not at all talking down to people who are in wheelchairs, and if that would have been my future, I would have made the most of it and figured it out. But to have my world flipped upside down in an instant was jarring, to say the least, and for a fifteen-year-old it was world shattering. In this instant, my brain was in an angry survival mode—in a good way. I was determined—and inspired by Dennis Byrd. I was persistent with the physical therapist about getting me out walking. I kept pushing it almost to an uncomfortable end, but it worked. She eventually agreed to work with me on walking a little at each visit, *if* I could walk three tiles with her walker.

The walker was blue, like Duke University blue. It wasn't a regular walker, but kind of a hydraulic lift. It had four little wheels on the bottom of a U-shaped structure. Out of the base of the U was the pillar that came up to another U-shaped structure with padding. Both U's opened up toward me. On the back of the pillar was a pump. She wheeled the walker up to me and told me that I could hold onto the pads while she lifted me out of the chair. The deal was that if I could walk three hospital floor tiles she would teach me how to walk.

Thirty-six inches. I was running hundred-yard sprints a few days ago, and now my future of walking relied on me moving only thirty-six inches. As she rolled the walker up to me, I thought it would be easy. Three little tiles. I was cocky if nothing else, and angry—and at that moment my anger over Dr. Beard telling me I would never walk again and then dismissively walking out of my room was fueling me. His beady little eyes flashed in my mind. I could say "fuck you" to him and everyone else if I could walk these thirty-six measly inches. Easy, right?

I was set. She started pumping the walker up. I could feel the increase in pressure on my forearms, and my grip on the pillar increased with each pump. I could feel my torso and abdomen start to tighten like it did when they tried to lift me off the couch at the beginning of this whole thing. Still to this day I get spasms in my abdominal muscles when I go from sitting for too long to standing straight up. It still almost always pulls me downward, a reminder to me that I need to keep working to stand up and keep moving forward.

After seven pumps the pressure on my arms was maxed out and I could feel my legs start to move under me. And instantly, doubt and fear hit me. I struggled to even get my legs underneath my body—how was I going to walk with these legs? Then the anger came back again, almost as quickly as the fear. I *couldn't* let them win. I would walk thirty-six inches if I had to drag my legs with me.

And that is pretty much what happened. I thought it would be easy, but it felt like I was at the end of practice running hundred-yard gassers in the August heat. I remember each ugly waddle of the thirty-six-inch runway to my goal. It was not pretty, but white knuckles and all, holding the handles as hard as I could, I made it. I was strong enough with my upper body that I was able to kind of waddle the whole thirty-six inches. I had bruises on my forearms and probably lost some skin from the vinyl pad rubbing as I used all my upper body to move my weak and pathetic legs.

Someone followed behind me with my chair the whole thirty-six inches (must have been grueling for them, ha-ha). I hit my goal and collapsed back into the chair behind me, huffing and puffing like I just completed a 5k. It wasn't pretty, but I made it. I had fulfilled my half of the bet, and my therapist would eventually fulfill hers as well.

After getting Natalie on my side, getting up and ready for therapy became like getting ready for football. I would approach it the same way that I would get ready for practice. The only difference was that my goal wasn't to win Friday's game but to walk a couple inches farther than last week, or to lift my arms and stand unassisted for half a second longer. If I could complete each week's goal, I would get to my ultimate goal: walking. Walking was my Superbowl.

Therapy was kind of like *The Karate Kid*. I would get frustrated at the activities because all I wanted to do was walk, and I didn't see how such simple exercises were helping me get there at all. One of the therapies tested how well I could use my core to control reach. I had to move a pile of stuffed animals and weighted balls from a chair on one side of me to an empty chair on the other side. It was difficult, and seemingly pointless, so I got frustrated with it.

I asked Natalie why we were doing something so stupid. Just like how Mr. Miyagi prepared Daniel for karate with seemingly meaningless tasks, she was doing the same with me. She explained that even though it seemed pointless and tedious to pick up the little objects and move them side to side with control, it was part of the bigger picture.

I want to walk, and to walk I have to swing my arms. If my arms are swinging, they will be adjusting my center of pressure, so my core has to be strong and coordinated. I needed to build that foundation before we could work on the actual walking.

Once I understood that, it was on. I pushed myself harder. I had to build my core. It was a struggle at first just to lift the different animals and weighted balls, but eventually I got good at it. In order to push myself, we would move the tables farther and farther away to force more movement and better control of my core.

Building the core is a principle that I now always try to impart to my patients. I can hear my mentor and friend, Dr. Michael Hall, in my head with this one too: *axial before appendicular, balance before coordination.* You see, learning to walk mirrors many things in life: we must first have a strong foundation, a good base, before working on the more peripheral things. I understood this, again, in football terms. Good teams build in the trenches first. Make a good offensive and defensive line first, then develop the skill positions. Even though the running backs and receivers get the touchdown, nothing happens if you aren't good in the trenches. My therapist quickly made me understand that I needed to be good in the trenches before I could do the flashier stuff—like actually walking.

I never thought in a million years that I would have ever called walking "flashy stuff." So many things I had taken for granted, so many little things I had to retrain my body how to do. For example, at fifteen I never thought that I would have to relearn getting on and off a toilet. While I approached physical therapy like training for football, occupational therapy was approached much differently. OT meant working on basic skills, the activities of daily living. It wasn't harder from a physical standpoint, but it was definitely harder from an emotional standpoint. Working on things like toilet transfers were totally necessary, I get it, but they were also kind of pathetic from my point of view. It was hard just to think about the fact that I actually needed to work on these simple things. In my mind, I wanted to be so far past this stuff—besides, my plan was to walk out of the hospital, so why would I need to work on transferring from my chair to a toilet? Many of the other OT tasks seemed tedious as well. We would do puzzles and other "fine motor" tasks, as well as upper body gross motor. I remember getting so bored on the arm bike. I would fatigue out, yes, but if I was being honest it was just because I didn't want to do it anymore. Knowing what I know now, I wish I would have taken that training more seriously. The things that they were working on were more specific to the brain than they were to the body, and they would have helped me greatly in the long run. As a kid, I really just wanted to push past all of that.

Each day was a new challenge, but once I got my mind right there was improvement almost daily. I remember a lot of the little victories, like being able to stand with the walker for the first time, being able to wiggle my toes, and getting in the parallel bars for the first time. That was a big one. The parallel bars are exactly what you are probably thinking of—if you have ever seen the Olympics, they look just like that, only lower to the ground. These two metal bars were placed two to three inches above where my hands were with my arms comfortably by my side. They were intended to give me something to hold on to as I walked my way between them. You have probably seen this process done in a commercial or two. Usually on TV it happens with someone who is learning how to walk with a new artificial limb. The bars are ten feet long and you still use your upper body to help you walk, but it doesn't feel as pathetic as the walker. The walker has a stigma around it that you are old and frail. Think about it—that is normally who you see using a walker, right? It has a way of quietly demoralizing you but is still a necessary step in learning to walk.

Unlike the walker, the parallel bars were actually fun. At first, the therapists were right on top of me with a gait belt—a belt that went around my waist for support. But once I got comfortable, I did a few dips and pretended I was training for the Olympics. The bars gave a sense of freedom while standing and walking that I hadn't had with some of the other tools.

I was walking. They told me I'd never walk again, but here I was, *doing* it. I needed the bars, but I was getting better every day, and before long I wouldn't need the bars at all.

It would have been the easy way out for me to accept a wheelchair, and if I had, they would have taught me to use the chair and released me from the hospital with some fancy new wheels. Not because they are bad people but because the system is a machine and the doctor's words are taken as bond. They don't see the possibilities; they just see the case that was laid in front of them. They have to check boxes and get to a certain number of people because there are always more people waiting for that hospital bed. Unfortunately, it is up to the patient or their family to advocate for themselves and see what the possibilities could be.

Never accept your new normal.

It is easy to listen to what they say and to feel down about your diagnosis, and it is perfectly normal to allow yourself some time to grieve and feel bad. Doing that for a little while is healthy but lingering there too long can get that emotional limbic brain wound up. Then you become your disease and have trouble seeing past it. When we live in our limbic brain, we steal blood and resources from our frontal lobes and cerebellum, the two areas of the brain responsible for rational thought, seeing the big picture, and keeping our thoughts and emotions balanced and coordinated.

So, go ahead and wallow for a minute. Then, after that, get off your ass, turn on your frontal lobe, and figure out how to fix your problems. Or call someone to help and give you some hope. Hope can be a powerful thing. With hope, I have seen people overcome some seemingly insurmountable things.

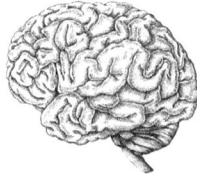

CHAPTER FOUR

Biggest Triumph and Failure

My most triumphant day was also the day of one of my biggest (and to this day, one of my hardest) falls. It was after training in the parallel bars. As I said before, the parallel bars were one of my favorite exercises. It was one of the only times during treatment that felt like I was doing an actual workout. I also got to work with one of my favorite therapists, Dr. Moon, who was a former football player, like me. He had a similar story to mine, too—he also injured his neck playing football.

Tears welled up when he told me his story. He described how, during a game, he was going over the middle to catch a pass. As he crossed, he could see the linebacker drop into his hook zone, and as he saw the ball leave the quarterback's hand, he knew it was going to be a high ball. So, he jumped in the air to get his body into position to catch the ball, but also to take the hit from the linebacker that he knew was coming. He said he remembers feeling the ball hit his hands...then the next thing he can remember is looking up at the coaches and trainers as he came back to consciousness.

One of the trainers was holding his head and the other was asking him to wiggle his fingers and toes. He remembers feeling relieved when they said, "OK, good." In his injury, he got pinwheeled and landed on his head. What that means is when he went up to catch the ball, his lower body got hit and he spun and landed upside down on his head. He lost consciousness and ultimately fractured his neck. He was in the hospital for a while too. He had to heal from the fractures in his neck. He had to go through a lot of physical therapy to get back his quality of life. Hard work and perseverance allowed him to get back to being healthy. It ended his football career, but his healing journey put him on a new path: working with other people who were hurt.

He used his lowest point as fuel to get him through school and through the physical therapy program. It brought him to a rewarding career of helping people find their own motivation and to push through their injuries. Just like he had persevered, he could use his tragedy to help others get through theirs. I didn't realize how much his story would drive me at that time. All I ever thought was, "This guy gets it, and if he could do it, so can I."

Damn, this book is hard to write through the tears sometimes...

Dr. Moon would always push me, to get me to do more than I thought I could. A little bit of fear would instantly creep up when I felt his pressure from the belt around my waist decrease. As I could feel more pressure on my legs, I was sure I was about to fall, and I'd grip the bars really tight and stop until I felt all was right on my foreign legs.

After a couple really good sessions back to back, Dr. Moon challenged me and let go of me completely a few times. I was able to string together movements that began to look more like actual steps as I made my way down the bars. *I'm ready*, I thought. *If I can make it, I will be home soon.*

Before long, it was time for me to try to walk the whole length of the bars at once with no help. As Dr. Moon told me how it was going to go, I was getting excited. It was only ten feet, but at that point it was like completing my first marathon. In my chair before getting up, I was psyching myself up in my head, like I would before a play when I knew I was getting the ball. I ran through the checklist in my head of what I had to do and mentally rehearsed each step. I was thinking about hand placement and challenging myself to keep from using my hands at all.

Before I got up, I remember thinking, *If I do this without my hands at all, I'd really impress everyone.* I'd have them there for balance, but I planned to not put any weight on them. I rocked in my chair and pulled myself to my feet, using the bars for support as I steadied myself.

I could feel Dr. Moon behind me as he said, "You can do this, but I'll be right here if you need me."

I had to rock myself a little on the first couple steps. I worked cautiously and slowly, making my way. I could still feel Dr. Moon behind me, but in my head, I was getting farther and farther away from him and closer and closer to leaving. I could see my dad to the side of me and hear his words of encouragement, too. Finally, I made it to the end of the bars with a big exhale. I don't think I took a breath the entire trip. As I got to the end, I looked behind me and saw Dr. Moon had followed me with my chair. I asked him to take it back and began my turn around. I wanted to walk back, too.

Dr. Moon smiled and said, "Alright."

I was invincible. I had just walked ten feet and I wasn't exhausted. I knew I could keep going. With each step back, I felt like my gait was smoother. It actually felt like *walking*. I only used the bars for reference on the way back. I was flying high.

I had finally made it, I was healing!

I collapsed in my chair for a break, winded a little after the trip back. I could kind of feel the blood pumping through my legs, like after a tough workout on leg day. It was a great feeling.

The bars were the end of the day's therapy session, and I was on top of the world. I wanted to push my wheelchair back to my room on my own. I had this vision of looking normal, walking down the hall pushing the chair instead of sitting in it. I remember thinking that I was finally better. I could finally see the light at the end of what seemed, at times, like an endless tunnel.

Filled with confidence, I stood again, and I started walking toward the automatic door in the PT room. I felt it was a journey out of there for the last time.

I made it about ten feet, then collapsed under my own weight. My legs were so fatigued—I had underestimated the toll all the exercise had taken on me. At first, I couldn't believe that I was laying on the ground. Then, in a flood, the feeling of triumph was gone, replaced by that darkness of the endless tunnel. The white hospital tiles were cold on my hands and forearms. I didn't want to look up at Dr. Moon or my dad.

I had just made everyone so proud, and now how would they look at me? How much had I let them down? Was I ever going to get better and get out of there? My dad pushed me back to my room. I kept my head down in defeat, fighting back the tears until I was in the privacy of my own room.

Moments like these are when you really need people in your corner. It was easy to go back to my room and sulk and feel like

I was never going to get better. People were telling me things like "Don't worry about it, you still had a great day in therapy" and "You did so much that your legs were just tired." But as I heard those words, I just felt worse because people had to make excuses for me. However frustrating they were, those words were also the only thing that kept me going (after I got done sulking, that is). When we feel the most isolated, having those around us who care about us can pick us up the most. Even when, at the time, their words may be the last thing we want to hear.

Therapy is tough. Don't let anyone tell you different. It will challenge you, both mentally and physically, every day. Some days, you wake up motivated and ready to take on the world, and others you will want to keep hitting the proverbial snooze button. The therapist that I had was great and she liked to push me, but some days I had to make sure that she was pushing me. After two or three sets of the exercise where I had to move stuffed animals from one chair to the other, I reached down and pushed the tables farther away from me to give myself more of a challenge.

Natalie laughed and said, "Sorry, I wasn't pushing you hard enough today."

Some days, you have to figure out how to make things harder for yourself and push, and other days you have to dig deep just to get out of bed. It is important to do things to push yourself and the people around you, even as the patient.

I have seen both sides of it now. As the doctor, I know it can be easy to fall into a routine with a patient. I am fortunate to work with other doctors in our office. I can always have someone else work with my patient for a while as a fresh set of eyes, or I can pick someone else's brain for new therapies. I always have my neuro-nerd friends on speed dial to call if we get stuck on something for too long.

If you are a patient, do not be afraid to speak up and ask about switching it up. Sometimes we don't even realize we have fallen into a rut. In a hospital setting, there are always a lot of therapists and techs to help make things interesting, so make sure you are taking advantage of that.

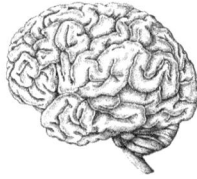

— CHAPTER FIVE —

ROOMMATES, FIELD TRIPS, AND LIFE IN THE WARD

It is hard staying in a hospital for a month, especially in the Neuro Ward. One of my roommates was a man who was unconscious in a coma the entire time that we were together. He just lay motionless in the bed, never making a sound except for the beeps of the machines that he was hooked up to. Most of the time, however, you couldn't hear the sound of the machines over the cries and apologies of his girlfriend who stayed by his side, holding his hands faithfully. I found out through overhearing some conversations that he was there because of a horrible car accident. He and his girlfriend were heading home late from a concert. She fell asleep at the wheel and drove them off the road, down an embankment. While she escaped with only minor injuries, ever since the accident he had been unresponsive to the world around him. Her guilt weighed so heavily on her that her face had what seemed like permanent tear stains on her cheeks. She would only break from crying for brief periods, and that usually was to pray for him or to continue apologizing. It was difficult to see and feel the emotion in the room. It made me realize that what I was going through was bad, but there were harder cases in the bed right next to me, and I should be a little grateful for that.

My next roommate was further evidence of this. He had been in a bad horse-riding accident that had damaged his neck so badly it severed his spinal cord. He couldn't breathe on his own, but he was conscious. When he would talk, you could see his pain from the machines helping him breathe—or maybe from the positions he was lying in. At night he would groan and make these weird coughing noises in his sleep. His agony made me realize again how bad it could be. Despite my terror, confusion, and depression, at least I was never in agony like this man. When he was awake, he was surprisingly upbeat about his condition. Even with all his pain, he was determined to get out of there and walk again.

My time with all my roommates was relatively short, and I don't know what became of any of them, but their imprint on my stay, healing, and life after my time in hospital has been profound. Sometimes they come back to me in nightmares of cries of sorrow or agony mixed with the beeps of life support. Other times they come back to me in the strength I pulled from their journeys to realize that mine could have been much more difficult. And finally, they come to me in the lessons that I learned from their journey that led them to be my roommate. I still can't really sleep in cars and have a lot of trouble being a passenger. My wife and I joke that I need the control, but I think the opposite is true for me. I would never want to see anyone feel the sorrow that I saw that woman go through from having made a simple mistake. I would rather take that responsibility, knowing if anything ever happened, it would be my fault. I don't only attack driving with that mentality, but everything I do in my life.

First Field Trip

My first field trip out of the hospital was about a week after being let in. They let me go to the hotel that my dad was staying in. It wasn't a big trip, but I was excited to get out of the depressing walls that had surrounded me. I had been in therapy for a while now, so I was able to help get myself in and out of the chair and onto the bed and things, so I wasn't a complete burden. When we got to the room, the first thing I wanted to do was take a bath. I wanted to just sit in the tub, instead of being wheeled into the shower and sprayed down. I was very excited to just rest in the water.

Being in water, whether it be pools or lakes, was always my happy place. This was no pool or lake, but at least I would get to just sit and relax in it. After filling the tub, my dad helped to get me down in the water. It was great to just sit and soak.

I had only been in the hospital a little longer than a week, but the atrophy in my legs was significant and jarring. I felt shocked the first time I looked down at my shrunken, shriveled legs beneath the water. It was frightening. It was really the first time I had looked down at them straight without something covering them.

How could this be? Only a couple weeks before, I was in top football shape. I was squatting a few hundred pounds and running and jumping—and now, looking down at these pathetic excuses for legs, it was surprising that they could even support my own weight to do a chair transfer. It is amazing how fast the body can learn to do new things, but also how quickly we can deteriorate without the proper signals from our nervous system.

Without nerves feeding my muscles, I had wasted away to almost skin and bones in the matter of a few days. My once mighty legs that propelled me down the field now looked like twigs.

That is how a lot of things were in my healing process: one victory (getting to leave the hospital) followed by a defeat (realizing how shriveled and pathetic my legs had become). It was tough trying to muster the energy to get through each of these events. Sometimes I found myself stuffing down my excitement because I was waiting for the other shoe to drop. I still do this at times. But you have to push through. You have to.

Through this process, you will realize what the human body and mind are capable of. How amazing things are. You will learn to appreciate the small victories but not get washed away in them either, so you can get back to work and keep pushing forward. This was the mentality that I had to adopt to get through things in the hospital.

This was the first time I remember hearing about the 90/10 rule. Life is 10 percent what happens to you and 90 percent how you react. If I had allowed all the little things to affect me the other way around, or even 50/50, it would have driven me into a deeper hole I would not have been able to crawl out of. I learned, with that mantra and with each negative thing that happened to me, that I had a choice to respond with self-pity or to respond by using it as fuel to drive me forward. Everything began to look like a challenge that I had to conquer to build myself up. It was not something that was being done *to* me that I had to wallow about, but something that was being done *for* me to sharpen my skills and take me to the next level. Sometimes it can be hard to dig deep, but this gave me some extra motivation, when needed, to push through. The 90/10 rule became my mantra, both in the hospital as well as when I returned home.

Dr. Beard and His Bedside Manner

I have really tried very hard to let things go pertaining to this injury and all the things that have happened, and for the most part I think I have done a really good job of it. Writing this book has helped immensely. But, no matter how hard I try, I still have some anger towards Dr. Beard and the way that he treated my situation. It wasn't the information he told me, that I had had a stroke and would (likely) never walk again. As a doctor, I know that when we run tests we are comfortable with, we read the results of those tests as we know them. He was reading his tests his way, and he came to what was a solid diagnosis for him at that time. So, I don't fault him for the diagnosis.

What I *do* fault him for is that, as a doctor, we swear to an oath of "do no harm," and I do not believe that delivering news like "You have had a spinal stroke and you will never walk again" with a cold, callous, heartless approach abides by that oath. To take hope away from someone, especially so early in the process, does harm. Maybe not in the form of a visible scar or bruise— it doesn't bleed or cause swelling, but it is potentially the most damaging injury that a patient can receive.

Those words were an injury to my frontal lobe, the part of the brain that sees the big picture and thinks past the problems in front of us to figure out solutions. By dashing hope, he decreased activity in the part of my brain that could have helped me heal the best.

Now I am not saying doctors need to be all sunshine, rainbows, and unicorns. When you have to deliver bad news, you have to be stern and direct in delivering it—however, there is a right and wrong way to do that. We can still be stern and direct while still giving hope.

When doctors approach patients as a number or just as the condition—or worse, a collection of symptoms or test results—it dehumanizes the case. I get why doctors may think this is a good idea. It allows for some separation from the patient so as to not get too attached. That way, if something goes wrong, the doctors can maintain that emotional distance and not get too wrapped up. It is one of the first things they teach residents in school, how to separate emotionally and not get attached. This will allow you to move from patient to patient, applying the knowledge you have obtained from years of studying to the set of symptoms and test results that lay before you.

Removing that emotion or that connection is a big problem with our health care today. Now, I am not saying that all doctors need to be emotionally invested in their patients' health and take on their pain or suffering, but there is a way that we can be emotional and compassionate to our patients without getting too attached. There is a way for us to look at them with honesty in our eyes and convey that there is hope that they can get better. I am also not saying that we need to tell every patient that they will completely heal and get back to normal. We do have to deliver hard information and facts sometimes, but that information doesn't have to come with a frigid demeanor that offers no room for hope.

Yes, our science may say that circumstances are dire. When we have seen this condition in the past, *this* has been the result. However, we can also choose to report what the *other* small percentage of patient outcomes have been. If a condition has a 1 percent success rate of getting better, let's focus on that. Let's get the patient's brain working on that possibility because the hope that they could be the 1 percent is what might be the thing necessary to get them there.

The brain and the body are remarkable. We really only understand a small part of both. There is always room for the miraculous, and there is always room for hope. And with the speed of research changing our understanding of science and health daily, who's to say that we won't figure out a way tomorrow to heal what is impossible today?

Another Field Trip—Sometimes, You Just Need to Laugh

Field trips were always awesome. Getting out of the hospital and back into the real world made me feel human again. One time, my mom and Aunt Angie took me out for some real food, to get a break from the normal hospital feast. We went out to The Golden Chopstick in Traverse City for some Chinese fare.

In northwest Michigan at the time, Traverse City was the biggest city around. Even though it was seventy miles away from my hometown, Manistee, it wasn't abnormal for families to make the pilgrimage up to Traverse City for a day of shopping, since the city offered the only mall around. So, as usual, The Golden Chopstick was packed with families and kids trying to get something more substantial than what the food court offered.

Anyway, while we were waiting, we heard a guy getting angry. Apparently, the host was not giving him the answers that he was hoping for in regard to the timing of his food. It wasn't long before the manager was coming to the aid of the poor high school girl that this guy was laying into. The manager was not any more help.

The whole thing ended with this guy erupting at the top of his lungs, "I want my four egg rolls! I've been here for an hour, and I want my four egg rolls!"

He repeated this over and over as loud as he could for several minutes. The whole restaurant froze, at first, and stared at this guy losing his mind over four egg rolls. I remember getting pissed, at first, at how he was treating the people he was yelling at. Then it was just hilarious. The people in the restaurant who had originally frozen in surprise started snickering and pointing. Even the manager was fighting back laughter at this guy as he continued his rant.

Finally, a staff member hurried out from behind the bar and apologetically handed a take-out container to the man. He stopped, huffed a little more, and then retreated to the parking lot, four egg rolls in hand.

The door wasn't even closed behind him and you could hear the snickers coming from the tables around us turn into giggles. Even the manager and hostess were having a laugh at the gentleman's response.

Now, I am not judging him or what he did at all. Who knows—he could have been having a shittier day than I was, maybe a shittier month. He could have been in Traverse City with a family member in the hospital down the hall from me. There are a whole host of things that were probably going on in his life, but was screaming at the staff the proper way of handling it? No.

Maybe he gets a pass for whatever he was going through, but whatever caused his distress, for me it was the first really good laugh that I had in a long while. Maybe since before getting to the hospital. It was a welcome reprieve from all the crap that had been running through my head. For a minute, I was just a kid with my mom and Aunt Angie enjoying Chinese food. For a minute, it felt normal, like how life was before. For a minute, I got to forget that I was in a wheelchair. It was a great break from everything.

Laughter and jokes would prove to be a necessary distraction. Laughter and friends and family were a big part of keeping my spirits up and realizing I would get through it. As Patch Adams said, "Laughter is the best medicine." It definitely was an important part of my recovery. You have to learn really quickly not to take yourself or your surroundings too seriously. You need loved ones and friends there to keep it light, keep you laughing at yourself and the crazy guys at the restaurant. If you can laugh at it, you are closer to beating it.

That event in The Golden Chopstick is still a running joke with my mom and aunt. I don't think I have gotten Chinese food since that time without that story popping into my mind, even for a brief second.

Needing Connection in Your Time of Need

This was the hardest thing I have ever been through. Even though it is now also one of my biggest motivations, other parts of it still sting. However, as much as I talk about it being the hardest thing "I" ever went through, I think it was equally hard on my parents and family. I know for a fact that without the support of my mom and dad I would not have been able to make it through the way that I did.

My mom was the first one who came to me when I woke in the morning unable to move my legs or feel anything, and my dad drove five hours north and was at the hospital before I even remember coming to. They both helped me in ways that I can never repay.

My parents were divorced when I was three years old, so I don't really remember them being married, but they always got along in front of my brother and me. They never seemed to let their differences get in the way of my brother and me feeling loved and cared for, and this event was no different. They say you really find out what people and families are made of when things are hard, and that really rings true for me and my family. I was really lucky to have parents as strong as them.

They were both always there for me in their own way. My mom was always the motivator and the one pushing me to strive to be better in life, so she was always pushing me in the hospital, too. My dad, in contrast, was always the one who let me vent and get stuff off my chest. He always knew when I didn't necessarily need a pep talk or to hear that I could do it but rather needed to be pissed or pout for a minute. I definitely needed both of those approaches at different times when going through all this.

The things we go through bring our family along with us, whether or not we plan for or realize it. We can and should draw strength from the fact that people care about us and are willing to be there to help us. Draw strength from their support in different ways, and draw strength from knowing you are not alone, even at your lowest point. Those around you are there to pick you up. It is very easy to retreat into what you see around you. So much sickness and illness can become your reality. When you are down and out and living in a hospital, never underestimate how important it is to have a connection to the outside world, to healthy, happy people.

Having people visit was very uplifting, but also hard. I remember telling my parents that I did not want my brother to come to the hospital. I did not want him to see his older brother broken and defeated. It was hard for me to see my friends, team-mates, and coaches for the same reason. My coach was a huge man, strong, a prison guard at the maximum-security prison in our town, and someone I admired. He pushed me to succeed on the field. A few days before I was a warrior on the gridiron, but in the hospital, I was a weak, frail, and scared kid who didn't know what his future held.

In the end, despite my embarrassment, it was key to have those people visit. Having friends and family and being connected to a bigger group gave me strength. Even though I didn't want my friends and family to see me the way I was, it was supremely important for my recovery to have them around. We all need that interaction to heal and be healthy. Knowing they cared made all the difference in the world. Feeling like a part of a team gave me a purpose: to survive and strive again.

The prefrontal cortex needs movement to be healthy, and it also needs social connection. Our brains actually *require* interaction with others to be healthy. The connection to others and something bigger than yourself, like a team, can give us purpose beyond just survival.

The Blue Zones by Dan Buettner discusses how scientists identified a few areas in our world that had the largest concentration of people who live to be one hundred years old. The areas were Okinawa (Japan); Sardinia (Italy); Nicoya (Costa Rica); Icaria (Greece); and among the Seventh-day Adventists in Loma Linda, California. The biggest difference from the rest of the world that these areas had was not their diet, air quality, or climate, but their social structure. These communities all knew their neighbors and had conversations with them daily. They felt like they were part of the community and that they not only had a responsibility to those around them but that those same people had and honored a responsibility to them, as well. The science shows the importance of having people support us, and I know that for my journey it was hugely important to have something even bigger than my family (though I do think we sometimes take family for granted) that I could belong to. Having that responsibility to others sometimes gives us the power to heal.

At some points, when I felt like I could just give up, I remember thinking that my teammates would have pushed me. Coach wouldn't have let me quit. Being able to pull from that allowed me to dig deeper.

The other area that I pulled a lot from was the responsibility of being an older brother. My brother was always a great athlete, but even more than that he was always the hardest worker on the field. Growing up, my brother was a little overweight and would get picked on for that. I watched him use that as fuel on the field as we grew up and in the weight room in the off-season. Before long, he transformed his once pudgy body into a brick. He was unstoppable on the field as a fullback, and the last thing you wanted to see coming through the hole when he was playing middle linebacker. I simply couldn't quit on him. I couldn't give up and return home weak and frail. I had to set the example, continue to work, and get back up and walk out of here. This gave me that extra motivation. It wasn't the first time I would draw on my relationship with him for strength and it definitely wouldn't be my last. Responsibility and connections to others fuel us.

Even something as simple as getting a small present from someone is enough to lift your spirits. I remember getting an actual mixtape from my cousin Lisa (for those of you too young to remember, a tape was a way to listen to and record music. Before Apple Music, MP3, and even before CDs there was the tape). She had put all sorts of, looking back now, pretty dark music. It was my first exposure to artists like Pearl Jam, Pet Shop Boys, and Smashing Pumpkins, and it kind of became my soundtrack while laying in the hospital. You can only watch so much daytime TV as a teenager until you start to go numb, so I would listen to her tape on repeat. It wasn't even my type of music, but I thought that I should listen to it because she made it for me and, in a way, that made me feel supported by her and my family. In my time of need, something as simple as her mixtape was very meaningful to my journey.

I actually like some of that music now too. Lisa opened me up to a new genre, but more importantly gave me a connection that I needed to heal.

There are a few mementos from my time in the hospital that I still have and cherish. They were mementos that showed me support in my time of need, symbolizing love and care. My coach, Coach Pant, came up to see me in the hospital and brought me some magazines to keep me busy. He also brought me a football that was signed by the whole team. I still have the football. It has moved to five different states with me and is still one of my most cherished possessions. It has written on it our overall record of 5–3–1. The "1" was my last game. Very symbolic how the only tie game I was ever in as a football player was the game that I was injured in.

Being in a small town as a teenager has its downfalls—it can be pretty hard to get away with things when everyone knows who you are and where you're supposed to be—but it has a lot of positives, too. Like how when you are going through something really hard, the whole school rallies behind you. At least, that was my experience. Another souvenir that I still have from my time in the hospital is a giant banner that was signed by everyone in the school with wishes for me to get well. Nothing motivates you more knowing you have a few hundred people in your corner to support you and cheer you on. It is crazy what will motivate you in hard times. I might have thought something like that was cheesy in another circumstance, but at the time it was a prized possession. It still is.

I am not and never have been a very religious man. I believe in a higher power, but I am just not sure that any one religion has it exactly right. However, I was raised Catholic by my mom and especially my grandparents. My great-grandmother had one picture hanging in her house that always resonated with me. It was the footprints poem. When I read it after my injury, it brought tears to my eyes.

In the poem, God is talking to a man in heaven who is looking back at his life. The man asks God how come, if God is always with us, there are sometimes only one set of footprints in the sand, especially during the hardest times of the man's life? God replied back that he hadn't abandoned the man, but instead, "my son, that is when I was carrying you."

That hit me really hard.

I was drawing strength from everyone around me—my parents, my brother, my friends and family, coaches, etc. But something in the universe was helping too. I seemed to have an endless supply of "get it done," and for that I am thankful to that higher power. That is one of the big things that I look back on with my injury to show that it wasn't done *to* me but *for* me. The universe put that obstacle in front of me to make me the man I am today and to show me how to be stronger and how to overcome. Something was carrying me when I needed it most, and I thank my great-grandmother for unknowingly hanging some inspiration in her home.

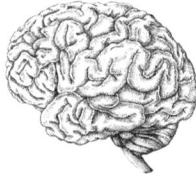

CHAPTER SIX

MY FAMILY'S JOURNEY THROUGH THIS

What became apparent, while writing this book, was that my journey was not just mine. It also affected those around me. So, I asked my mom and dad to tell me about what it was like for them. My mom teared up when I asked, but that made me even more sure that I was on the right track. If she still teared up that easily, the wound was still fresh to a certain point. My dad had a similar reaction. It took some time, but they were able to write their perspectives on the event. I hope that it gives some insight into how the shared journey is experienced from different perspectives.

A Letter from My Mom

I don't think I will ever forget Michael's scream. I can still hear it. He screamed, "Mom!" in such a way I thought he was in pain. Michael wasn't in pain—in fact, just the opposite. He couldn't feel anything at all. He couldn't get to his feet, and he couldn't move his legs, only his arms.

My younger son, Chris, ran next door and got help. When we couldn't get Michael on his feet, I called an ambulance for help.

Manistee Hospital couldn't figure out what was wrong, so they called a neurologist in Traverse City. Michael was taken in an ambulance and I followed behind in my car. They wouldn't let me ride with him. I remember being pretty numb. When things start happening and you can't deal with it, I believe you just react by putting one foot in front of the other. Must be some kind of survival instinct.

The neurologist ordered an MRI, blood tests, and all sorts of other tests that I hadn't heard of. I worked in health care with other doctors for over ten years, so I was somewhat familiar with the medical world, but I still didn't know all of what they were doing.

This doctor may have been one of the best in his field, but he knew nothing about dealing with people. He told me Michael had either had a spinal stroke or multiple sclerosis, but at any rate he probably wouldn't walk again. I thought, *What?!* Are you crazy? He's fifteen, what are you talking about?

I called my sister Angie. She wasn't able to understand me because I couldn't stop crying. Hours later, they finally put Michael in a room in the children's ward. After Michael got out of the children's ward, they moved him to the neuro floor. There we met a gentleman that had fallen off a horse and broken his neck. I don't remember his name; he had been in the hospital for weeks.

This man gave us lots of encouragement, and told us not to give up, ever. Michael changed rooms a few days later and the man gave me one of his plants. Said he wouldn't need it, he would be walking soon, even though the doctors told him he would never walk again.

I still have the plant; it has been with me since that day. I will have to remember to give Michael the plant someday so he can care for it. The plant, for me, became a symbol. I had to keep it thriving and healthy. It's my oldest plant, and it is still going strong. Like Michael, the plant has adapted to its surroundings as I've moved and it has done well—actually, it has done great. Like Michael, it's a true survivor.

Weeks and weeks of physical therapy followed. It was difficult watching my son suffer so much. I would have traded places with him in a heartbeat.

On one outing, when he was in crutches, I picked Michael up and they let us go out to eat and come back to the hospital later in the day. While going to the car, Michael fell, but the stubborn, determined young man refused assistance from any of us and got back on his feet and crutches by himself. Of course, we laughed with him just so he knew how much we loved him—because it was heartbreaking!

A Letter from My Dad

I remember the football game. Thursday night. After the game we went out to eat. You were complaining that your back hurt then, at the restaurant. Next time I saw you, you couldn't walk.

Mike, I'm having a hard time writing this. It still hurts. Your mom called around ten o'clock a.m., and she told me when you woke up that morning you could not walk. They took you to the hospital, and the hospital transferred you to Traverse City. Your mom and Mike (stepdad) gave me directions to get there, and Sharon and I just got in the car. I do not remember the ride up there.

The doctor came shortly after we got there. He told us he thinks it was either MS or a spinal cord stroke. He wasn't sure which, but he told us either way, you would probably leave the hospital in a wheelchair. Your face went blank for a couple of days after that news.

I drove home to get some clothes and money and arranged to take time off of work. When I got back, the doctor told us he believed it was a spinal cord stroke. He was going to treat you with steroids and physical therapy. Your mom and I told him you would leave the hospital walking. After a couple days of physical therapy, you were standing and walking a little bit.

Your mom talked about transferring you to the Mayo Clinic in Minnesota. We talked about it and I thought you needed to be close to home and friends. Visits from your friends and teammates seemed to pick up your spirits. Your mom and I figured we could have you checked by other doctors later, if you needed it.

One day I went hunting with your brother Chris. When I got back to the hospital later that day, Sharon was pushing you outside in a wheelchair. You told her to stop and you got out of the wheelchair and walked a little way toward us. I didn't stop smiling all day after that.

All that I can remember about the day you left the hospital is that you left walking. I knew it was still going to be hard for you, but you were walking.

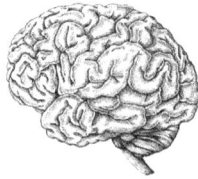

CHAPTER SEVEN

LEAVING THE HOSPITAL

I remember the day I got to go home like it was yesterday. I was so excited. I was returning home. I wasn't one hundred percent yet, but I was much better. I had some difficulties, but I would get rid of them just like I got rid of the ones that I had with each challenge in the hospital.

They sent me home with bilateral crutches and a cane. They were talking about my physical therapy that I would need to continue to do in the hospital near home. You remember the place that sent me home with a pain med and muscle relaxer? The journey would come full circle by ending where it had begun. I would need to allow that local hospital to have control of my health once again.

It was a little bittersweet, leaving the hospital. On one hand, and it is a really big hand, I was free. On the other hand, I was about to enter a world that wasn't controlled. Everything was easy in the hospital; I knew what each day had in store for me. I had a regular schedule and knew where I needed to be at all times. More importantly, I knew everyone there and what they thought of me—well, this version of me. The version that still couldn't walk too far without having to take a break. They saw me through the hardest time in my life, so I had a little trouble leaving those people behind me, especially for a situation that was so uncertain.

After the initial excitement of getting out, fear quickly crept in. The little devil on my shoulder started to speak loudest, asking questions like, what is everyone going to think of you? How will you be treated? What if you can't make it to class, or fall, or worse yet, you lose control of your legs and all strength and have to be carried or wheeled somewhere? For a brief minute before being let go, I wanted to stay. The reality and uncertainty of the situation got really real, really quickly, and what was a very happy and exciting event had a little fear to accompany it.

Knowing what I know now, I think every big event is a little bit like that. If it really matters to you, there is definitely excitement. If it really matters to you, there is also, at the very least, a little bit of fear to go with it.

What I remember most was actually leaving the hospital. I was able to walk on my own—I had to use a cane, but I was able to walk. As they worked on processing my paperwork, I remember standing there with my parents, proud of myself that I could stand, excited to do what I had been dreaming of for weeks and walk myself out that door.

Then one of the orderlies walked up with a wheelchair. At first, I thought they might be there to get someone else, or maybe it was a joke. It wasn't a joke, and it *was* for me. I tried fighting with them and told them that I would walk out on my own. Was this some kind of reminder that I was still broken? I *earned* the right to walk out of here. For me, walking out was my triumph. The moment after the doctor told me, on that first day, that it was not possible for me to walk out of the hospital,

I had been planning this moment as my big "fuck you" to the doctors who had put limitations on me. How could they think I would be alright with this? How could they want to take this away from me?

But it was hospital policy. They would not let me walk out. No matter how much I begged and pleaded with them it wasn't going to happen. It was a "cover their ass" policy in case I fell or something on my way out. No matter how much I told them I would be fine, they would not budge. The compromise was that I would sit in the damn wheelchair to the front doors, then my family would pull the car up at the bottom of the drive and let me walk from there—with my cane, of course. One more hoop to jump through, whatever. I was out of there and on to new challenges.

The Return Home. More Challenges

Getting out of the hospital had been my goal for so long. I would lay in the hospital bed and imagine being able to go home to get up and change the station on my radio, to go see my friends, to just listen to quiet—since at home there were no buzzers going off at all hours, and no nurse to wake me up just to give me something to help me sleep.

I had all these visions in my head of the things I wanted, but I hadn't really prepared for the challenges. Like, how was I going to get around school? Wait, *school!* I had missed over a month of classes. Even though some teachers had sent me some of my schoolwork, a few of my teachers didn't send any and told me I could make it up when I got back. I surely had a mountain of work waiting for me. There were all sorts of things I *needed* to do, after I got past the things that I *wanted* to do.

In addition to working my way back into school, I would also have to find time to make it to outpatient physical therapy. Even though I was mobile now, I was far from "back." My legs were still really weak, and my balance was pathetic. Long gone were the days of being able to run or jump. It was a struggle to make it a city block without having to take a break. But I was free, back on my own terms and in my own house.

It was great being back at home. I was able to do all the things I had hoped for, and the quiet was amazing. I was finally able to lay in my bed, stretch out, and be alone with my thoughts.

At first it was comforting, to be able to hear myself think. But when you are recovering, and not as fast as you want to, your own mind can be a dangerous place. The silence was great until doubt about ever being completely normal started to creep in. This is, again, why it is so important to have that support system. My friends were great at allowing me to feel like I could fit back in. They helped me get around, and especially helped me to feel normal again by getting into trouble, like teenagers do.

You know the joke that goes: How do you tell your best friend from a good friend? A good friend will bail you out of jail if you get in trouble, but a best friend will be sitting next to you in the cell. That best friend for me was Luke. Luke, Brian, Denny, Ty, and really too many others to name, made me feel like me again. Most importantly, they didn't treat me like I was broken.

After getting home, I had a few days off before I had to go back to school to kind of get acclimated to life outside the hospital again. It was nice not having to jump right back into things. When I left the hospital, the physical therapists had given me hope that some of the lingering symptoms would get better slowly. They told me to look out for little things, like tingling in my legs or feet, or the ability to feel temperature in extremes. Both were signs that things might be starting to wake up again.

The big question for me was how long I would have to use a catheter. This was my biggest fear about returning to society. It was weird and gross to me, and I had had a month to get used to it—how would my friends look at it?

The doctors told me that if I had an accident while I was sleeping, or even while awake, that may be a sign that things were waking up down there, that the nerves were starting to have a better connection, and I might be regaining control. Well, it happened. The night before my "welcome home" party, where my parents invited some friends over to the house to see me, I woke up soaked.

I was over the moon excited.

Yeah, that is not a normal reaction to that event, I get it. And yeah, I know that sounds *really* fucking gross, but this meant the end of having to use that damn catheter. What might seem disgusting was actually one of the most exciting things to happen to me in a while. After getting cleaned up, I asked my mom to immediately call the hospital and ask what it meant. I asked her to ask them if I could stop the catheter. They were happy to hear me so excited, and they said that I could try. They warned me not to get too excited, but I was so happy the one thing I was dreading the most was something I might actually not have to worry about.

I tried not using the catheter for the day as friends started to show up. I still had no feeling down there, but I had faith that something would happen if I needed to use the restroom.

It was great having friends around before going to school. It was easing my fear about having to go to school because I got to see everyone on my turf first. It seemed a little normal, hanging out with everyone in the basement and playing video games. Talking with everyone and catching up on all the high school drama that I had missed over the last month made me feel more like myself again.

It was only about an hour into the party when my hand brushed the crotch of my pants on accident and I felt it. It was wet, and I was mortified. I used one of the blankets from the couch to cover myself. What was starting to ease my tension was now starting a panic attack. The ease of getting into conversation now turned into me nervously trying to keep everyone talking so that I wouldn't have to change position and expose the disgusting truth.

I never even felt it. I have no idea how long it was like that before my hand noticed. I couldn't feel it on my legs or anything. What if that happened at school? I would never be able to go back. A new fear had surfaced, and this one was a big one.

When I called the hospital back and described what had happened, they said it was normal, but something I would have to monitor myself. Not only would I need to continue manually emptying my bladder, but I would need to stay on top of it so I would not overfill and spill out.

Being back in school, at first, I got all the looks—all for good, of course. People were happy I was back. I am sure there were more than a few rumors as to what had happened to me, too. Especially in high school, that is the job of some students: to create rumors. But everyone was very accepting and welcoming, and that was huge. After the initial stares of disbelief and wondering over how I was walking, it all calmed down. It was great to be around friends and support again.

The highlight of my return to high school was my visit to the last varsity home football game against Benzie Central. It ended up being a 19–8 victory for our Chippewas over the Benzie Central Huskies. As much as it was a highlight to be back down on the field, it was also a little weird. Because of liability, they had to wheel me down onto the field, and I had to promise to use the crutches to get around on the field. It was also weird because I wasn't standing on the sideline with my Junior Varsity team—but it was still cool to be there. Some of the guys that I looked up to came over and said hi while I was standing there with the crutches. It was nice to stand on the sidelines again. It gave me a sense of being home.

Physical therapy had given me a few rules that I was supposed to follow. They wanted me to not push myself and to take it easy, which meant walking with a cane, but there was no way I was doing any of that. None of that was how I got out of the hospital in the first place. I get that they were just looking out for me and trying to cover their own asses, but I was never going to roam the halls with a cane. I actually did take it with me to school every day, mostly to keep my mom from nagging me about it. I would carry it the whole way to my locker, hang it on one of the hooks, and that is where it would stay until classes were done. And to "not push myself," I took the elevator and had people carry my books for me. The thrill and popularity of having the elevator key wore off pretty quickly. I was taking the stairs and pushing myself almost immediately. I am sure that they saw that coming at the hospital though. I wouldn't slow down while I was at the hospital. There was no way I was going to slow down once I escaped.

It was great having friends to support me and having the school rally around me. Even with the difficulties of using the bathroom and having to fit in time for physical therapy, it was a very supportive environment. However, after going through something like this, I was different. Experiences like this change you. At fifteen, I was supposed to just have to worry about homecoming dances and being cool. There is supposed to be a certain amount of innocence, but all of that changes when you go through something like this.

I knew that some people out there had it much worse than I did. There were kids starving on the streets and going through abuse, and those things are all horrible, but for me, this experience was the worst.

Suffering is relative.

That is something I tell my patients to this day. I might have a patient who has a memory issue sitting in the waiting room next to a guy who is in a wheelchair and can't feed himself. The person with the memory issue almost always starts their visit by saying something like "Wow, I should just suck it up and get over it. I don't have it nearly as bad as that person."

Yeah, maybe you don't have it "as bad" as someone else. But when we are going through something, I think that it is important to get the opportunity to feel bad for yourself for a minute. You need to allow yourself that feeling of the world being against you. You need a little "woe is me," but don't allow yourself to wallow in it for too long. Don't let it become you. Feel it, then get over it and use it as motivation. Use it to dig deep and pull yourself out. It is all relative, and what you are going through should not be minimized by someone else's issues, even if you perceive them to be worse than your own.

For me, this was as bad as it could get. And it did change me. I found it hard to listen to my friends' stories about how bad some things were. Now, I know that sounds hypocritical because I literally just got done saying that it is all relative, but it's true. I just didn't think that their struggles were that big of a deal most of the time. While they were telling me their problems, I always thought, in the back of my head, "Hey, it could be worse. You could be paralyzed. Get over it." It was easier to blame it on them, but it was me who had changed.

Because of this reaction of mine, this lack of understanding of the phrase "suffering is relative," some friendships changed and grew apart. It was hard to take at first. Growing up that much, that quickly, is hard.

I think the universe gives all of us only what we can handle, even if it doesn't feel that way at times. There really is no growth without struggle or suffering. If we were all just coasting along in life, we wouldn't be improving, growing, or changing.

What someone else is going through does not minimize your suffering. I know that it is human nature to compare ourselves to others around us, but we need to separate from that mentality. What we are going through is *our* journey, what *we* are meant to overcome. Just because it is different from someone else's journey does not make us unworthy of feeling the weight of it.

It reminds me of one of my favorite posters. It depicts a scene from the 2016 Rio Olympics when Michael Phelps, an American swimmer, won five gold medals. In the picture it says, "Winners focus on winning and losers focus on winners." You see Phelps hyperfocused, looking forward to his goal. He was just a little ahead of the onlooker, Chad le Clos, a South African swimmer, who was trash talking Phelps before the games started. Le Clos is looking over at Phelps, not looking ahead to a strong finish. When we focus on what others are doing around us, it can take away from our journey, from our drive. It detracts us from focusing our energy on attaining what it is that we need and want out of life.

If we *can* take one lesson out of comparing ourselves to others, though, is that we should not think our weight is too heavy to do anything about. Meaning, if we look at another's journey and see the heavy load they bear on their shoulders, we can realize our rock is actually not too heavy to push up the mountain, since they're doing it too—and sometimes, they're doing it under even harder circumstances. It can sometimes give us the confidence needed to conquer a task. I know I just spent a few paragraphs telling you not to compare your journey to that of another person, but if doing so gives you strength, not weakness, use it. If your meaning comes from understanding that what you are going through isn't that bad and that realization gives you motivation to push past it, use that as your fuel.

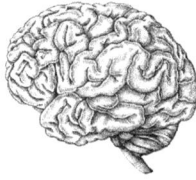

— CHAPTER EIGHT —

CONQUERING FEAR

The act of pushing through something harder than I ever thought possible was a big part of my growing up, but another very big part came from contemplating death the way that I did. I didn't tell anyone until years later, but the first couple days after the doctor told me I would never walk again were dark. Very dark. Going from playing football with friends and dreaming of maybe making football my career to all of a sudden being told that I would never walk again was shattering.

It made me really think about how unimportant I was to the world, and I wondered if I really did bring much more to the table than my physical talents. I cognitively knew that I was smart, and a good person, and all that junk, but my biggest asset had always been my physical ability. Without that, what was I? Emotionally, I was broken. When you are in that state of mind, the limbic brain really puts you into survival, fight-or-flight mode and actually takes blood and resources away from the logic parts of your brain. This decreases your ability to make rational thoughts.

I thought a lot about what I was losing, and this caused me to spiral down pretty quickly. My limbic brain was thinking in absolutes, and I absolutely thought I needed to end my life. This wasn't teenage angst. It wasn't a fleeting thought of, "Well, then I'll just kill myself." I had a lot of time to lay there and really plan out how I would do it. If I couldn't walk and play football, then I felt my time here was done. I rationalized that this was a sign from the universe that it was time to go. I had plans of how I would say goodbye to everyone that I loved. How I would explain to my friends and family in letters that this was best for everyone. How I didn't want to be a burden to my family. How I didn't want them to have to take care of someone in a wheel-chair. I was very ignorant at that age and had no idea what kind of plan I was meant to fulfill, and I didn't really care. I just knew I didn't want to burden those I love.

I started feeling better about life during physical therapy, and when Natalie agreed to help me to walk, I stopped consid-ering suicide. However, I knew I would keep feeling depressed until I conquered sports. Ironically, sports terrified me. If I was going to conquer sports, I would first need to get my body stron-ger and improve my stamina. With how weak and frail I had become, the thought of being in the weight room with my old teammates was intimidating. Knowing how far I had declined in physical fitness; I was ready for the long road ahead.

Getting over my fear of sports was hard. I say "fear" because I know now that is what it was. Even once I could walk reliably without the cane, I couldn't play football. That was obvious. I was still weak, way too weak to be an athlete. I couldn't even bench one hundred pounds for a long while. I was scared that I would never be able to do it again. I was scared that many of the things that I loved to do and that defined me would never come back. I still went to physical therapy every day and to the weight room after that, but it wasn't the same. It was just me against the weights, and a lot of times the weights won. Every time anything would feel weird, it would scare me. I missed the camaraderie of the team and feeling like a part of something bigger than myself, but even as I regained my strength, I was too scared to risk another injury.

One time I was doing back squats after school. The place where I had to rest the bar on my back was very close to the area that was damaged in my spinal cord. While I was lifting, I felt a pain in my spine. It was foreign for sure. I didn't have feelings in my back or from there down at this point, and that pain scared the shit out of me. I racked the weight slowly, making sure not to let the pressure off my spine too quickly. I slowly took my weight belt off, scared that any little movement might cause something to break. I then slowly walked out of the room and down the flight of stairs to the main floor of the school, where I gently sat down on a bench in the hallway, and even more gently lay down on my side. The whole time my senses were on high alert for any sign or symptom that my injury was happening again. I don't know how long I laid there but it felt like forever, silently listening to my body for anything that would indicate a problem, wiggling my toes every once in a while, just to make sure I still could.

After a while of not having any other kind of symptom or tingle or trouble breathing, I slowly sat up and tested my legs on the ground. After ensuring my legs could support the weight of my body, I stood up, walked to the staircase, and proceeded to walk up the stairs again, testing to see if my legs felt heavy or hard to move. They didn't, and after getting to the top of the stairs I let out a big sigh. I was clearly just freaking out.

I would learn something in school as an athletic trainer years later. We always said that an athlete's body was ready much before his mind. Meaning, when rehabbing an athlete from an injury, like an ACL reconstruction or meniscus or any other sort of injury, the injury was healed before the mind was ready to trust it. I was no different. I would need to trust that my body could do things that it may not have been able to do before. I needed to know I really was able to get strong again.

After a While, Things Start to Feel Normal Again

After the normal day-to-day started to fall into place, things started to look normal. A different normal, but normal, none-theless. The amazing brain, in order to feel comfortable with new surroundings, adjusts and falls into a pattern really quickly. My new normal included the fact that therapy replaced my gym time and sports. Through workouts, I was able to control my bladder better, too, so the catheter slowly phased out as I gained more muscle control. Fatigue was also getting better. The more I walked, the more I could walk. I seemed to fade into the background a little more at school, too. I was catching up on my classes and I no longer drew sad looks from people as they walked by. It was nice. I started to feel a bit like myself again.

Now don't get me wrong—I still had quite a few things that separated me from my classmates, but for the most part they were not openly visible to the naked eye, so people viewed me as "normal" again, and it was nice.

Some of my continued deficits were actually kind of fun. I still hadn't regained the perception of hot and cold from the waist down. I couldn't tell by feeling it, but my body would give me signals. For example, when getting a shower ready, I would dip my toe into the tub. If it was too hot for my legs, my leg and foot would jump, kind of like bouncing. We call it *clonus* in neurology. The legs were more sensitive than the hands, too.

Something that wouldn't feel too hot on my hands might make my legs jump uncontrollably.

This seemed like a real bummer at first—but there is always a bright side, right? The bright side for a junior in high school who is just discovering parties and beer was that I could hold a lighter to my leg longer than anyone else. That earned me more than a few free beers before my friends caught on to me. Growing up in the country, we had more than our fair share of bonfires in the woods, too. This new superpower allowed me to firewalk without pain longer than most, as well. Except for Garrett, but he wasn't right in the head.

The downside to this lack of temperature perception is that this feeling travels on the same system that perceives pain. Now, not feeling pain sounds great off the bat, until you stub your toe in the middle of the night and can't walk. You see, my body didn't feel the pain, so it found other ways to let my brain know there was an issue. If I had anything happen to my legs, I would temporarily lose the use of that leg. A stubbed toe was no longer just a quick flash of pain to walk off. Now it was a long, drawn-out loss of function of the affected leg until my brain could figure out that everything was OK. Then I had to walk it off until the leg felt normal again. Sometimes it could take two or three minutes to regain the complete use of the leg.

A story from my wilder days of self-discovery is one that happened pretty early on in high school, while out at a party in the middle of the woods. This was no different from a usual party, except for the fact that someone had brought pallets for the bonfire. Pallets are fun because they burn really quickly and get the fire roaring, but they also provide a platform for ignorant teenage boys with beer to test their manhood. Do you see where this one is going?

It was my turn to test how long I could stand on the pallet that was just placed in the fire. This was pretty late into the party, so the fire was nice and hot by now, but this only upped the ante and impressiveness of the feat. We threw a pallet on the fire and climbed on after it, cargo shorts and all. I knew I still couldn't feel pain or temperature, and with a few beers obstructing my judgement, I was planning on going for the record.

Standing in the middle of the fire with my arms raised, screaming like an idiot, was pretty easy at first. I could feel the heat making my chest sweat, but nothing in my legs. The next heat I felt was around my cheeks, like when I got too close to the fireplace at home. After that, it got unbearable because even though I didn't have feeling in my legs, the face was working just fine.

I decided to jump off, but unbeknownst to me the fire had reached the pallet that I was standing on and was burning through it quite a bit. As I squatted to jump off, the pressure caused my leg to push through the partially burned boards of the pallet. Now my foot was squarely *in* the fire, and I was up to my knee in the pallet. My reflex was to scurry off the fire, dragging the pallet, wrapped around my shin, with me.

I had cleared out a ten-foot circle around the fire, kicking up quite a few sparks and flames in all directions. I was fueled with adrenaline, but the odd part was that there really was no pain. I could feel a little pressure and could not put weight on the leg with a second-degree burn, but no pain. The fear of the situation set in pretty quickly though. I smelled the burned flesh and realized that my foot just didn't look right. With all eyes of the party now on me, all I could do was shake it off, literally, and plunge my lower leg into the nearest cooler. There was a hiss when the burn met the cold. Thankfully, the owner let me keep the cooler for the ride home until we could get dressing for the wound.

Every time I think of that story, I remember the song by Garth Brooks, "Standing Outside the Fire," and every time I hear that song I think of this story. The song uses the fire as a metaphor for the struggles of life. Fools who need to take chances constantly continuously reap the negative consequences of their actions. The strong, who seemingly don't need any help, can brave the journey on their own. The weak are the ones who never seem to take chances and never push for their dreams. The line "those without scars have lived safe and maybe have never really lived at all" (Standing Outside the Fire, 1993) has always stuck with me. I always looked at being weak as one of the biggest insults. However, sometimes taking crazy chances can be foolish.

I think we are all each of those people at different points of our lives. For a while I was weak and I did forsake it all in the pursuit of trying to feel something good, something that would compare with the high of learning to walk again but that would also drown out the low of knowing I would never be the person I was before. I was definitely foolish when standing in the flames too long, almost losing myself in the process. But the lesson from that moment allowed me to understand when it was right to stand strong and stay out of the fire.

Now, twelve years sober, twelve years out of an even bigger fire, I am on the path I was meant for. I was dangerously close to becoming foolish forever, but instead I was lucky enough to know when to get out of the fire before I was completely consumed by the flames. I learned the lessons that "living" taught me, so I could use them as strength to help others.

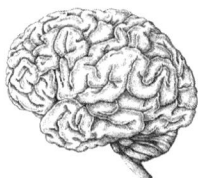

CHAPTER NINE

MY FIRST ADJUSTMENT, AND NEUROLOGICALLY WHAT HAPPENED

After settling into my deficits and learning to deal with them, I kind of got sick of second opinions. I was always hearing new things that might help, only to have my dreams dashed again. I had a few problems left that were kind of annoying, but for the most part they were not affecting my life to a point that I was willing to keep going to doctors all the time. I just wanted to move on and feel normal. I was done searching for answers. I just wanted to exist and hang out with my friends, like any other sixteen-year-old.

The father of a friend of my brother was a chiropractor in town. My brother had recently been to see him. I remember Chris telling me how much better his back felt afterward. He often had back pain from football and lifting—nothing serious, just the normal postgame injuries and muscle tightness. He told me about all of his bones cracking and releasing and how cool the adjustment was. It sounded a little crazy to me, but I did have some back pain from some of my PT exercises and all the muscles in my body starting to come back.

When Chris told me about his neck cracking, though, I was terrified. I had flashes of every action movie I ever saw where the guy would walk behind someone, twist their neck, and *bam*, they're dead. I was already paralyzed once—I think I'm good. But after hearing from Chris and from some of my friends who were still on the football team, I decided to try it. I was extremely reluctant, but at this point I had tried everything else.

My friend's dad said he was really only offering to help put me "back in line" after all the trauma, not to fix any of the problems directly. After I was realigned, we would see what my body would do with that.

The event was jarring. He was an old-school chiropractor; he picked me up and shook me out like a rag doll. Bones cracked I didn't know I had. And when I was done, I did feel a lot looser, and like I moved easier, too. I was sore but this was a different kind of sore. I was also standing up straighter. He proved that, with a little pre- and post-adjustment check, comparing me to a simple string he had hanging from a metal form in his office. He warned me that I would be sore for a day or two and sent me on my way. I enjoyed the new freedom of movement and left.

That night I was getting ready for a shower before bed. I ran the water like I always did and dipped my toe in to check for leg jumping. But then something weird happened: it felt hot. *It FELT hot!* My leg didn't jump, but I could actually *feel* the temperature. I dipped my toe in and out a few times to check the new sensation. It was a miracle. What the hell happened? The only thing I did differently was getting adjusted that day with Dr. Boehm.

I went back to his office to ask him about it, and he simply said some stuff about how the power that makes the body, heals the body, and some other things that went way over my head. I was just amazed to have the feelings of pain and temperature back. That superpower of not feeling pain or temperature was cool and all, and it saved me some beer money, but like any party trick, it gets old. I was happy to be rid of it.

Our brain works on a principle of GIGO: garbage in, garbage out. If you have poor information coming in, you are going to have a breakdown. This breakdown may be in the processing of the total information you can have coming in or a breakdown in the movements, thoughts, or emotions going out. With my injury, there was a clear lack of information coming in, and at first there was nothing going out, either. My movements, although much improved, still didn't compare to my preinjury status, so there was a definitive lack of afferent input or sensory information. The physical therapy did a great job of improving my ability to move and got me out of the wheelchair, but it wasn't the huge afferent barrage that was needed to change that central integrated state—or reset the nervous system back to factory settings, so to speak. I would need a bigger input into the nervous system to do that, and for me, a chiropractic adjustment did the trick.

Your body is chock-full of these little things we call receptors. You have receptors that receive light, called photoreceptors, in your eyes. You also have mechanoreceptors, receptors that pick up movement in your muscles and spine, and these are the receptors that are activated with a chiropractic adjustment. When a chiropractor puts their hands on someone, they are changing the way that they perceive their environment. When they then deliver the adjustment with intent, focus, and force, they activate the patient's mechanoreceptors to send a huge signal up to the brain. This signal is called an *afferent barrage*, and it activates the brain with a symphony of signals, pinging around through the cerebellum to the parietal lobe to the frontal lobes. It sends a wave of energy all through the system that improves the brain's ability to take in all sensory information.

This is what I believe happened in my case. When Dr. Boehm adjusted me, he sent a huge signal through my nervous system and brain that woke some things up. When this happened, he activated some little receptors on the cells, called c-FOS and c-JUN, altering protein synthesis in the cells of the brain and nervous system. What this means is that he actually changed the ways that my cells were responding to their environment. The chiropractor epigenetically changed my body, and my cells started to create better proteins that did their jobs more effectively and efficiently.

He effectively rebooted my system and filled up the tank, all at once. This allowed my brain enough energy to feel temperature in my legs again.

The adjustment given to me by Dr. Boehm used a bank of receptors to awaken the perception of sensation in my body. In the same way, we can wake up the brain in something like hereditary spastic paraplegia. An adjustment and neurological exercises can even help something like depression or anxiety, something that current research is just now wrapping their heads around. Your body has receptors all over it for a reason. We are supposed to use them. We are supposed to move and experience our environment in 3D.

When we do this, the sky's the limit. The only limitations we have are in our own thoughts. If we can get past our own doubt, we are limitless, our brains are limitless, and we have the ability to heal, grow, and evolve in ways greater than we can comprehend. That is why my mantra has always been to never accept your new normal. Do not allow people to put boundaries on the things you can do. Do not allow people to put boundaries on what you can become or how great you can be.

Giving people hope allows for healing to take place. So much of the current medical paradigm is to assign a name to the condition and the set of symptoms, then handing out a medication designed to alleviate the symptoms from said condition. They don't focus on the problem in the control system. When we identify the problem in the system instead of naming the condition based on a list of symptoms, we can then better treat the *patient* and support what they need to grow and heal instead of focusing on the *disease*. When you have hope, you can dream. You are not just stuck in survival. Focusing on the disease gives people a sentence; focusing on the person gives them hope.

Back on the Field

As things started to feel more normal and I was getting stronger and stronger every day, the topic came up at home about me playing football again. This was a big point of contention for pretty obvious reasons—well, obvious to me now, anyway. I was a seventeen-year-old now, and it was preposterous that my parents would be against me playing again. How could they tell me that I couldn't do something that I loved? Even though the last time I played I ended up in the hospital, that did not stop me from bringing it up every chance I got.

I would argue that I would be fine, and I would be careful, and their argument was always, "Dr. Beard told you that you can never play any sport again, let alone football."

After begging my parents for weeks, they agreed that I could play, but only if I could get a doctor to sign off on my physical. I think they thought that the physical would kill the whole argument anyway because Beard would never sign the document.

I knew Beard wouldn't sign it, but I wasn't going to Beard. Never underestimate the motivation and drive of a high school kid who wants something. I went to my family physician. I don't think I was *completely* truthful with him about my previous history. I didn't lie to him, and he did know my history, I just didn't give him *all* the details of my current symptoms. He signed the document, and I was home free.

It was great to be a part of the team again, and really great to play on the same team as my brother again. We had not been on the same team since we were in grade school. Then, we were both standouts. Now, well, at least *he* still was. Chris was one of the best on the team and played both ways. I was nowhere near the level I was prior to the injury, but it was great to just be out there again, playing with friends and not feeling like damaged goods. I didn't mind not starting or even playing on a regular basis. I was content being able to play and work hard in practice.

I still remember the first hard hit I took in practice. I think a few of the coaches probably held their breath until I got back up, but it was great. There was hollowness to the hit on my pads and then nothing, just a little bit of pain when I hit the ground. It was a feeling unlike any other, and it was awesome to feel it again. It was enough to feel like I had made it back to the thing I loved so much, even though it had taken so much away from me before. It made me feel like I had won. Football wasn't stronger than me; I was stronger than it. I had taken its best shot and stood back up.

The most vivid memory in my mind from that year was from our last home game. It was an away game in Muskegon. My coach had told me during the week to prepare to play more for our last game. I guess he figured he would give me a win, since it couldn't hurt the record having a tight end that ran a 6.5-second 40-yard dash (for those of you not familiar with 40 times, that is about the slowest on the team) playing the final game. I joke now that you had to time me running with a calendar instead of a stopwatch.

My brother played great. He would build on his success, and eventually go on to play in college at Olivet in Michigan. But *this* game was mine. This was my last hurrah, and my big win. I played my best at that final game. I walked off the field having conquered football.

The day after our last game I was called out of class down to the assistant principal's office. He was also the athletic director. As I walked into the office, oblivious of what I was getting called in for, I saw his stern disapproving face. I realized this would not be a social call.

"I just got off the phone with your doctor, Dr. Beard," he said. "He informed me that he did not clear you for football, and that you were in fact not cleared to play any sports. You will turn in your equipment and you will not be permitted to play basketball or any other sports for the remainder of your time in school here."

My stomach sank. I had my one big triumph, but that would be it. It was a blow, but a minor one. I had conquered football, and that is all that mattered.

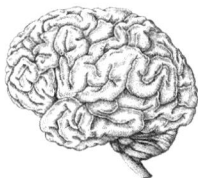

— CHAPTER TEN —

FROM FLYING HIGH TO CRASHING DOWN

My whole childhood I was obsessed with going fast. Some of my ability to do so was obviously affected by the injury. I had lost most of that fast-twitch muscle that helps with weights and speed, two prerequisites for football and sports in general.

Aside from physically running fast, I was obsessed with speed in vehicles, as well. I think every kid is enamored with fast cars like Lamborghini and Ferrari, and I was no different—but my real passion was in jets. I wanted to fly more than anything in the world. Before you think it, yes, I did see *Top Gun* too many times as a child, but we also grew up not far from an Air Force base and my parents would take my brother and me to see the air shows on a regular basis. It was always a game to guess the jets as they flew overhead when we were outside playing. I loved the freedom of flying around and the ability to go as fast as I could imagine.

That dream of flying jets led to a dream of being in the Navy and flying off of aircraft carriers, just like Tom Cruise did in the movie. So, when the military came to my school to talk to the students about a career in the armed forces, I was excited to talk with the recruiter about my plans. I was a pretty good student in high school. I was always good at taking tests, and even after the injury I was dedicated to physical fitness.

The steroids they gave me for inflammation had really done a number on me in the hospital. They ruined my complexion and caused some pretty extensive weight gain as well. Go figure—when you pump your body full of steroids and don't exercise, they still make you get bigger, just not in the muscular way.

At any rate, by the time I got to meet with the recruiter, I was thinking I was in pretty good shape. I had worked my body back, my mind was strong, and my eyesight (another thing I knew was necessary to be a pilot) was 20/20.

We started talking right off the bat about me being a pilot. I explained to him that I used to live near Selfridge Air Base down state and that I had been infatuated with flying ever since. He informed me that pilot was one of the most sought-after jobs in the Navy, but with my grade point average, extracurriculars, and physical fitness I could have a shot. Excited, I asked him about my next steps. He told me that in order to get into the flight program I would have to score really high on the Armed Services Vocational Aptitude Battery, or ASVAB test. I remember thinking, I got this, tests are no problem. He slowly slid the application for the test and test dates over to me, and while I signed my name he asked about my medical history.

I hesitated. He added that in order to get into flight school, I would have to be in perfect health. Not just physically fit, but I would have had to have been pretty much illness-free my whole life, too.

"We can't have someone broken flying a multimillion-dollar piece of machinery," he said.

My heart sunk. I got a little mad when he called me broken, but I knew I was sunk. I explained to him what I had gone through a little over two years ago. He looked me up and down and quickly pulled the application back toward himself.

"With an injury like that, I am not sure the Navy would have a spot for you, Son."

As quickly as he could pull the application back across the table, my dream of flying in the Navy was over.

My dreams were dashed, and this left me in a pretty dark place once again. I had sweated in the gym, at physical therapy, and worked my ass off to get back to normal, back to what my life was like before all of this started. I thought that I was past all this and that I would be able to return to my life as planned. For a little while, just a little while, I didn't feel like I was digging myself out of a bottomless hole. Not anymore. I didn't even have a backup plan without the Navy, at least not one that was feasible. I was pretty sure if the Navy would not take me with my injury history, then the FBI was probably out as well.

It is amazing how quickly you can spiral. When you lose your purpose, your goal in life, it is hard to keep everything on the rails. I had stuffed down a lot of defeated feelings in the process of pushing forward to my goals. But now, it was clear my goals were impossible. It seemed that all the struggle was for nothing.

In a small town there isn't really a lot to do to distract yourself from your problems. Your options are pretty much sports and drinking for leisure activities. Of course, in my town there was fishing, too, but that was about as exciting to me as watching paint dry. With sports off the table, this drinking thing was looking pretty fun. It allowed me to be fun and happy and the life of the party, and it took away about every bad feeling—at least until the buzz wore off. It was a great way to hold my sanity in place while finishing the last year of high school.

School was easy, so it wasn't hard to hold my grades down—plus, I pretty much had half the day off my senior year because I had positioned myself well in the first few years. But that was part of the problem. The extra time off during the day afforded me the time needed to take up smoking cigarettes and get really good at skipping the classes I did have. I was able to sleepwalk through the rest of school. I still got some sympathy from my teachers, so even if I did struggle, I was able to slide a little. Obviously, I had been through a lot, so I needed some leeway. It was easy to just keep my head above water and coast to a finish in high school.

I don't blame anyone for letting me kind of skate by, but I do give this information as a cautionary tale to parents and teachers of kids who are going through a lot. It is hard to tell when you need to let the kid be, and when you need to really ride them hard and make sure they aren't turning into a jerk. All of the people in my life loved me a lot. I know that now, and I knew that then. But I was hurting, and by that point I knew that I could use their love to get away with whatever I wanted. The desire to be numb to the world, the ability to get by anyway, and having enough people who cared enough about me to give me space was a toxic combination for me. I learned some valuable lessons in how to manipulate things to my advantage during that time (see above, how I managed to play football again). It wasn't a good lesson for me, but it was a lesson, nonetheless. In a small town, it was easy to let people see what they wanted to see.

But in between beer bongs and parties, I did manage to decide on a new path in life. Even though my previous plans had been dashed, I thought that I would use my experiences in life to my advantage (and soon, I would decide, to the advantage of others). After all, if the reason for the struggle wasn't to get my old life back, maybe the universe was trying to tell me to have a different life than the one I had originally planned for.

After looking into a lot of fields, I discovered athletic training. This would allow me to be involved with sports, even though I couldn't play anymore, and allow me to give back to others with sports injuries and help them get back on the field. My new mission would be to help others do what I couldn't do, to help others get back to their life even after an injury. After looking into a lot of schools, University of Detroit Mercy (UDM) was the best fit. They had internships with the Detroit Redwings and Detroit Tigers, and some Detroit team named the Lions, who I thought played football or something. My energy was renewed—I had a purpose in life again. I would use my struggles to help ease those of others.

In the next chapter of my life, it wasn't so easy to cover up my pain. It also wasn't so easy to coast by in college. At UDM, I was a little fish in a big pond. No one knew my history, but more importantly, no one cared. It was up to me to be in control of my own things and get my shit done. This was a slap in the face.

In the classroom, I struggled. My grades were way behind my usual standards, and I even ended up on academic probation. But however much I struggled with my classes, I excelled in the training room working with athletes. My good friend and eventual roommate Todd and I had been assigned a team of our own sophomore year, something that was usually not given until junior year. We got to work with the men's soccer team. The training room was great, and to top it off, my drinking and partying didn't cut into my performance there.

But it was not possible to keep up the drinking and the classwork. Instead of studying for a test or doing homework, it was easier to just polish off some Bacardi 151 (that is 151 proof rum. To put that into perspective, most vodka and other liquors are 80 proof). It was either that or Aftershock, a nasty cinnamon liquor.

One night I was in the computer lab—where you used to go to write papers before everyone had their own laptop or computer. All of my friends from the program had finished their papers, but I always waited until the last minute. I headed for the computer lab, bringing some Aftershock with me for the paper. It sounded like a good way to unwind and write. I never finished the paper, but I did wake up in a stall in the commons building with the taste of vomit on my breath at about four thirty in the morning. My friends had to come get me and help me get cleaned up. It was pretty embarrassing at the time, and I still have this pit in my stomach talking about some of those times now. I was having fun, but way too much of it. At the same time, I was still drowning in unprocessed emotions.

That sounds like a pretty low point, but it would get even worse at UDM. I don't want to turn this into a story of being down and out and turning to alcohol and drugs to ease my pain, but I do want to make a point that when not processed properly, your emotions can really get the best of you. They will affect you in ways that you are not conscious of and influence decisions that you think you are in control of, even when you're not. Pushing things down will only serve you for so long, but soon you begin to serve your emotions instead of the other way around. And when this happens, it is almost never good. When your emotions run you, you end up in a life that doesn't even begin to resemble what you had planned for.

I definitely spiraled for a while, losing control of myself and my emotions. It was like being in a haze for years, almost like being asleep and living a dream. Looking back at some of the things that I went through, I am lucky to be alive. I absolutely believe that I am only here because I have something I was put here to finish, and I am not done with it yet. After a long time, I realized that my journey, my struggle, was for me to help others. To understand how precious all the little things in life are and help others with them.

In our journeys, it is important to find meaning in the suffering that comes to us. Suffering is necessary to grow and to become a stronger, more complete person. When we lose that meaning and start to focus on only the negatives of what we are going through, that is when we falter. That is when we break down and give in to that negative voice in our head, which is run by fear. That is when we stop believing in ourselves. We have breakdowns because we don't have meaning. We have failures because we either don't have a clear enough goal, or we don't believe that the goal we have is attainable. As we make our goals or decide how far we can go, it is always necessary that our reach exceeds our grasp. Meaning, we should always shoot for the moon because even if you miss, you still land among the stars.

I made some great lifelong friends and unfortunately lost a few as well while working through my "detour" from my purpose. I met my loving wife while working at a bar during those times. Together, we helped each other on our journeys to reconnect to our purposes. After all was said and done, I would not change the past and what I have gone through for anything. As hard as it was, I would not be the person that I am today without having gone through struggles from my past.

I ended up on a journey that would have me working ninety hours a week *and* studying to get through school because my passion to help others had been ignited again, and by something that seemed so small at the time. A regular at the bar needed medical attention after he was hurt playing softball. Like it was second nature, I jumped up and utilized some of my training to get him taken care of. It was just an ankle sprain, but it was enough to spark that fire in me again to want to help others and get back to what I had set out to do leaving high school. It put me back on my journey.

This journey brought me to chiropractic school at thirty years old, determined to connect to a way of health care that was congruent with my beliefs. This journey saw my educational goals come full circle as I graduated valedictorian of my class. Most importantly, this journey reconnected me to the meaning behind my struggle.

Suffering is part of the journey, the way that we grow and find meaning.

We must find meaning from our suffering and have something in the future to look forward to. Victor Frankl wrote an amazing book called *Man's Search for Meaning* in which he recounts his experiences at a concentration camp in Germany during the Second World War. He talks about finding meaning in the suffering that they were going through and using that as fuel to get through each day. Now, if I had read that book before my journey, I could have taken it as a negative. Comparing my journey to his would have minimized what I was going through. My being in the hospital unable to move my legs would have paled in comparison to his trials in German concentration camps, but in his writing, he describes beautifully how taking meaning out of each of our sufferings led him to develop a new form of psychotherapy called logotherapy. In this therapy, he describes how they have the patient focus on looking for a reason to live because of meaning—that is, finding a goal or reason to be alive that is bigger than yourself. This is what drives us to succeed in life.

"Be aware of dissolution if your goals do not come to frui-tion but instead of seeing it as your meaning is lost, find strength in it" (Frankl, 2019). Reading this quote from Frankl's book smacked me when I read it. At one point in my life, I thought that my purpose was to be an athlete and then a pilot, but my injury unlocked a deeper meaning: one of service and of help-ing others find their new purpose and meaning. I realized I was meant to guide others' healing from the suffering that was put in front of them.

At this point I really like what I have become, and I work every day at not looking to the past and looking down on the events that happened to me, *or* for me.

Two more great quotes from Frankl that really stick with me in my life and that often come up in neuroscience:

> *"To be human means that we do not succumb to the reflexes and instincts as Freud might have said, but instead what drives us is our quest for a meaning and a bigger goal." (Frankl, 2019)*

> *"Man doesn't need equilibrium or homeostasis but instead exists because of striving and struggling for a worthwhile goal." (Frankl, 2019)*

These two quotes demonstrate the power of the human mind. The first quote is all about the frontal cortex. The part of the brain that separates us from the animals and allows us to see that we can get past the obstacles in our way.

The second quote is maybe a little controversial. In health care, we always tell our patients that we are striving for balance in the system. This balance is when your system is at harmony, or homeostasis. This may be the sweet spot that we are all aiming for, but just as perfection is not really attainable, neither is complete homeostasis. Instead of the constant search for balance, we may need to instead focus on the bigger picture. We are here for a reason. Whether you look at things from a spiritual perspective and ask, "What does my soul need to learn on this journey?" or from a more egocentric perspective and ask, "What will my legacy be?", we are all ultimately driven by meaning and goals. They are what allow us to ignore our animal instincts and become a part of something bigger.

Just remember: the obstacles that are put in your path are opportunities for growth and to become stronger, or to knock you onto a different path more aligned with your purpose on this planet.

Because of my journey, I will never take feeling the ground under my feet for granted. Because of my journey, I will always know how precious life is. Because of my journey, I know that no matter how depressed I get, there is always more to live for.

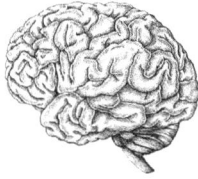

CHAPTER ELEVEN

MOVING FORWARD

It was years, however, before I woke up from the drunken stupor that I had been on. Years before sobering up, not just from the alcohol and other party favors, but also sobering up from the feeling of trying to control the situation and force my calling.

Once the alcohol wore off, I was able to think more clearly and perform better in school, but I was also able to hear more clearly the voice of something telling me what I could become if I would just follow the path that was laid out before me. What I could become if I stopped trying so hard to control the outcome and instead just listened. I was able to listen long enough to discover my journey.

However, it isn't as if that desire to control and manipulate things has gone away. That is something that was ingrained in me from a young age. "Work hard and you will reap the benefits," "God helps those who help themselves," and other similar self-help mantras that were the foundation for developing the young mind in the eighties and nineties still have a strong pull on my mind. The struggle to control things and people is still something that I must work on, on a daily basis. I especially work on trying to quiet my mind, and when I forget, I have my amazing wife next to me, shouting at me to get out of my head and just listen.

How This Affects Me in My Career

For a long time, I always talked about my injury as something that had happened *to* me, but at this point in my life I refer to it more as something that happened *for* me. It was a traumatic experience to go through, but it has made me who I am. I draw strength from it every day. It put me on a path toward working in health care and helping others who have suffered with similar issues. It gives me a purpose and a drive to be a part of something much bigger than myself.

I believe that the universe gives us what we can handle and challenges us to grow. For me, that challenge came early in life and was pretty big. I wasn't able to see it then—really, not until recently—but it changed me into the best version of myself. It took me out of a place of focusing only on myself and shifted my understanding of the world in a way that is hard to put into words.

I am now able to see the little victories in life better. Some mornings, just feeling my feet hit the cold floor beneath them is a win. I still get surprised sometimes when I put my foot in the shower and can actually tell that it's too hot. Every day, there are still little challenges from the injury—I'm not completely healed, even now—but there are also many little blessings from it as well. I always try to remind myself: it could be much worse.

I believe I have a little better understanding of where my patients are at, emotionally and physically, because at one point I was there too. I believe that my injury was done for me and for them, so I can help them through the journey they are going through. This empathy is something that I wish Dr. Beard had in him; his diagnosis may have been a little less traumatic for that fifteen-year-old to hear if it had been said a little softer. But then again, if he was empathetic, would I be pushing so hard to change the way health care is delivered now? Maybe not. So, maybe he was put there to drive me down this road as well.

The only real downside today to having gone through the injury is that I struggle not to "get in the pit" with my patients. I say this part because I want to offer some advice to anyone who may also be heading down this path, something I wish I had learned a lot earlier on. What I mean by "not getting in the pit" with someone is that I had to learn the difference between sympathy and empathy. A good friend and mentor, as well as an amazing man and doctor, Dr. Len Wisneski, told me once that I needed to have boundaries. He could see the toll that working with complex cases was taking on me. He could see the fatigue and frustration I was going through while trying to work out their cases and come up with answers for them.

He took me aside and told me that I needed to understand the difference between sympathy and empathy. "Sympathy is when you get down in the pit with the patient. You feel their pain and go through the journey with them. You even selfishly try to take some of their pain and help them get off their journey."

Selfishly?! What? I remember thinking. *I am the least selfish person out there. I am trying to help others!* Then I shut my brain up and continued to listen.

He continued, "Selfishly, you try to go through their journey for them. Would you have wanted someone to take your journey away from you? At this point, would you go back and give up everything that you went through?" I shook my head. My journey had gotten me to where I was, and I liked who I had become. "Then what right do you have to try and take their journey away from them?"

It hit me like a ton of bricks. I didn't have to—no, I couldn't *afford* to—wallow in their misery with them. It would drain me, as I tried to give them my energy to lift them up. I could not afford *sympathy*. But empathy *was* appropriate. I could be empathetic and help them and support them, but also challenge them to get up and move forward on their own. I shouldn't stop helping my patients or caring about them, but I should do it from a different place. That advice has changed my life, and it has changed the way I practice.

When working with people, empathy allows me to keep my energy up and still really dive into a case—but from the scientific end, to figure out what can be done neurologically and metabolically and so on, not from a place of wondering how I can take away their pain and make them "feel" better.

That was the difference for me. I wanted them to "feel" better. I wanted them to "be" better, too, but I was focused on trying to take away their pain. If someone had taken my pain away while I was going through my trial, I never would have made it out the other side. I know that now. And when I forget, I still have good friends and mentors like Dr. Gilles LaMarche and Dr. Wisneski to remind me.

This is another thing that my coaches and especially my parents unconsciously did really well for me. They did want to take away my pain, and at times they tried to. But they all also understood that I needed to get past my struggles, and that the only way that would happen was with hard work and by using my pain as fuel. My parents and coaches knew that athletes like me perform best with a challenge, when someone calls them out or tells them they are not good enough.

If you take it all in properly, it can be used for fuel that burns hotter than the sun. It can drive you over hurdles that you may have never seen yourself able to clear. When going through something tough, in order for it to really change you, you need a little pain. My patients need it, just like I did, to come out the other side.

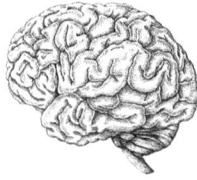

CHAPTER TWELVE

HEALTH CARE TODAY

I believe health care is at a crossroads.

The days of a doctor seeing you and dictating your health are over. The new generation is not putting their absolute faith in men with white coats, blindly taking their advice. With all of our new technologies, we have taken a peek behind the curtain and have seen the fallacy of the medical machine. Because of this access to health information at our fingertips, we have been given the ability to fact-check and be an active member in our health care journey. This new wave of ownership over one's health and the understanding that you really are limitless are working together to lead a refreshing health care revolution. And that change can't happen quickly enough.

Most Americans are currently taking at least one medication—or two, or ten. Over 12,512,000 children under eighteen years of age in the United States alone have been diagnosed with anxiety, depression, or another mental health condition and were given a prescription medication for that condition

(SAMHSA, 2019). We need to be questioning, active members in our own health, now more than ever.

Doctors are not bad people. They have everyone's best interest at heart, but with the burden falling on them to see more people, more quickly, they have to reach for the pad and pen to write a script more often. In fact, that is what is expected of them. Research has shown that many people value their visit based on whether or not the doctor prescribed something to them. Doctors are under pressure from patients who watch drug ads on TV and think they have all the symptoms, and they are also under pressure from Big Pharma, and both of these pressures have made it easy for pills to be their default. That, too, is why we need to be active. We need to research and understand what we are putting in our bodies, understand the recommendations of the doctor, and understand how they will affect us in every way. As a friend and teacher of mine likes to say, "There are not really any 'side effects,' just effects," and each drug can have a very different impact on different people.

It isn't the doctors who are the issue, but the medical machine that needs to be fixed. The paradigm shift is coming, and we need to take our own health in our hands. We need to know that we can get better. We may not realize it, but we actually have very little limitation when it comes to getting better outside of our own limitations of believing we can or cannot do so. After all, they call the doctor's diagnosis an "opinion" for a reason. The opinion they give is given with their filter; they are pulling from their experiences. Someone who has overcome seemingly insurmountable odds or has seen people heal from some pretty dire circumstances might have a different thought on the matter than someone with a more pessimistic outlook.

Perspective can make all the difference. For instance, in these two images, what do you see? In the first one, do you see a duck or rabbit? Can you see both? Do you see the vase in the second, or the two faces facing each other? How about the last one, an image once used to determine ageism? Do you see a young maiden or an old hag? These optical illusions demonstrate how the filter with which we see the world determines what we see. Someone with a different filter may see something completely different. Similarly, a diagnosis or prognosis is just based on perspective. They are not absolutes.

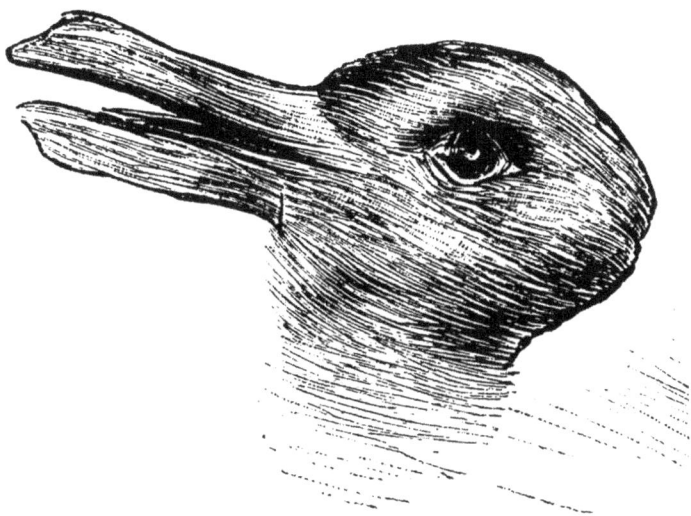

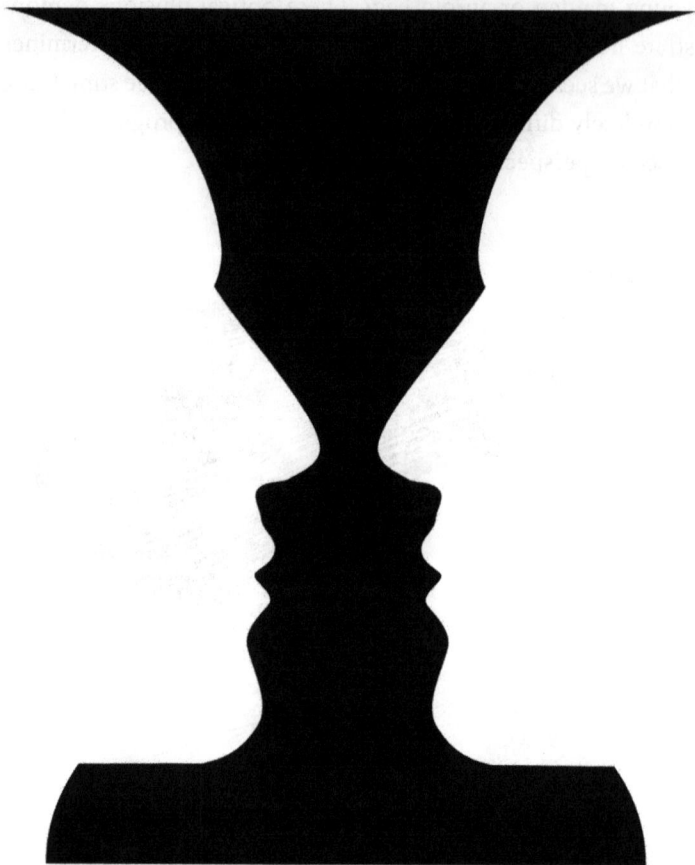

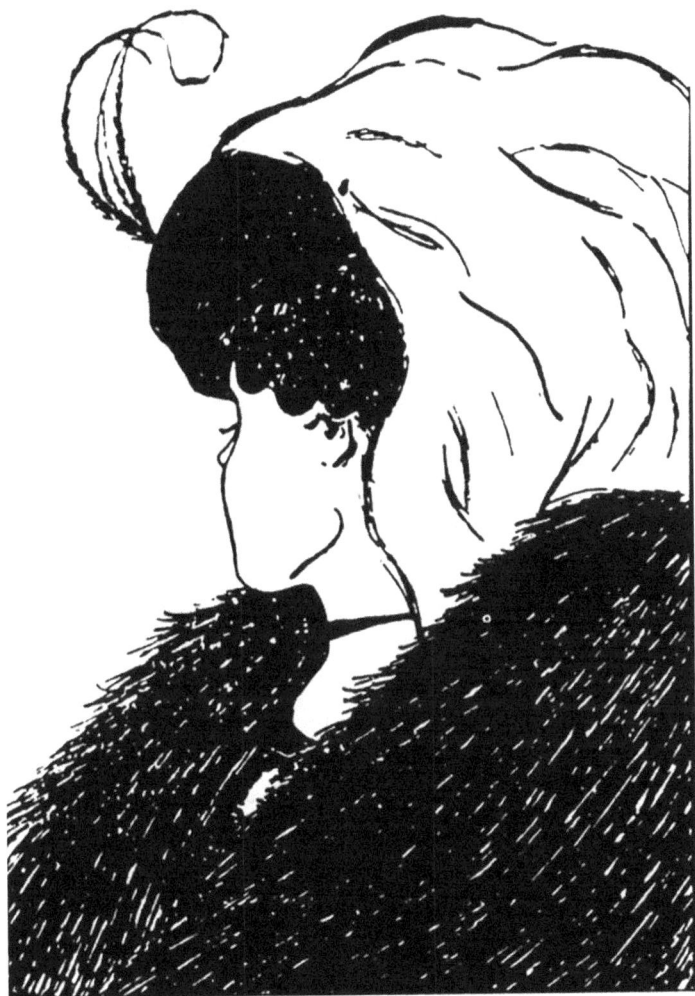

If doctors don't understand what is going on, they need to stop making the patient feel like they have no hope. Hope is a powerful tool. If the doctor does not understand where the patient is or what can help, they should focus on options that they have not yet explored. Just because a solution may be beyond our understanding does not invalidate it as a solution. Just because a solution is outside of our current perspective does not mean it cannot help.

As doctors, we often fall into specialties and ways of looking at things. If the person doesn't fit into that specialty or under that lens, we can't see the problem. We have had a lot of patients walk in our office with a stack of medical records who say something like "The doctor said that this is as good as I get" or "They can't find anything wrong with me to describe my symptoms."

A statement like "This is as good as you are going to get" is a bit ignorant. We really only understand a fraction of what the brain and body can do. To make a statement like that is limiting. The brain can do some pretty amazing things. I have seen things get better that are beyond my understanding, and that just speaks to the amazing potential of the brain and body. We should not put limits on it with our current understanding of neuroscience, medicine, or anything scientific.

Until the early 1900s, we thought the atom was the smallest particle—until we broke it open and found protons and neutrons and electrons. And we were sure those were the smallest—until we discovered quarks in 1964. Science grows by leaps and bounds each year, and our understanding of ourselves, the world around us, and even the whole universe changes almost daily. The power of the human mind to eliminate disease is just now being understood and is still largely untapped, so we should not discount the fact that the human mind can get us better. A further understanding of how our thoughts, perspective, and mindset really do control our health is imperative to move our current social paradigm forward.

Our current medical paradigm doesn't look at the body from the standpoint of what it needs to be healthy. It looks at the body as a collection of symptoms. Doctors then name this collection of symptoms and prescribe a chemical that is supposed to limit or eliminate those symptoms. There is no concern for health, just for the absence of symptoms.

We need to understand that the absence of symptoms does not equal health. True health does not come from a pill or tonic. It is a mindset, an active process that we are always striving for. We need to be conscious of what we are doing, eating, breathing, and thinking—*always*, not just when we have symptoms. When we do this and live this way, we allow the body's inborn intelligence to keep us healthy and functioning. When we use all of our senses to properly feed our brains, we develop a strong, healthy, and vibrant nervous system and brain.

With a strong nervous system and brain, we have the ability to adapt to whatever life throws at us. With a weak nervous system and brain, we are susceptible to diseases of the body and of the mind. When we cannot regulate our system, bacteria and viruses can more easily infect our bodies and depression and negative thoughts can more easily infect our minds.

In health care today, there seems to be a growing problem with mental health. This is supported by the numbers of mental health cases reported in the literature and unfortunately by the increase in prescription medications for things like depression, anxiety, and stress. In many cases, the treatments are just there to cover some of the symptoms for a while, and maybe even just to take the "edge" off. If the treatments don't work, the blame is often put back on the patient, and they are made to feel that their symptoms are all in their head or their own fault.

Our brain and nervous systems are responsible for controlling all of the chemical and biological responses to stress in our lives. When we push our brains and nervous systems too hard, they will start to break down. This breakdown will result in a change in physiology and function, and for some people this breakdown in physiology and function can manifest as cancer. It should scare us that the American Cancer Society reports an estimated 1,735,350 new cancer cases diagnosed and 609,640 cancer deaths in the United States for 2018 alone. There is a strong correlation in the literature that cancer is linked to stress levels, diet, and other environmental factors that we have control of in our own lives (Siegel, 2018). This all starts with our brains' abilities to control and regulate stress.

Heart disease is reported by the Centers for Disease Control to account for about 647,457 deaths in the United States every year, using the numbers from 2017 (Kochanek, 2017). That is one in every four deaths. Heart disease is the leading cause of death for both men and women in the United States. Every year, about 805,000 Americans have a heart attack (Benjamin, 2019). Heart disease has been very closely linked to lifestyle choices (Arnett, 2020). A regular regimen of healthy diet and exercise has been shown to be the most effective method of decreasing the chance of developing heart disease. However, diet and exercise alone will not work. Stress is also, again, a major factor in the development and progression of heart disease. Again, we know that having a healthy brain and nervous system is our best bet when it comes to handling the stresses of our day-to-day lives.

So, mental health issues, cancer, and heart disease are all known to affect a very large portion of our society. We are very aware of these conditions and the effects that they have on ourselves, our friends, and our family. We have cancer walks and heart disease runs on a regular basis—and these are all necessary because these conditions are debilitating and affect such a large part of our population. But, did you know that mental illnesses are even more common in the United States than these diseases? In fact, the number one reason for a prescription in the United States is for mental health. Nearly one in five U.S. adults live with a mental illness—44.7 million Americans in 2016 (SAMHSA, 2017). Mental illnesses include many different conditions that vary in degree of severity, ranging from mild to moderate to severe.

The National Institute of Mental Health recognizes two broad categories that can be used to describe these conditions: Any Mental Illness (AMI) and Serious Mental Illness (SMI).
AMI encompasses all recognized mental illnesses.
SMI is a smaller and more severe subset of AMI.
In 2016, there were an estimated 44.7 million adults aged 18 or older in the United States with AMI. This number represented 18.3% of all U.S. adults.
The prevalence of AMI was higher among women (21.7%) than men (14.5%).
Young adults aged 18-25 years had the highest prevalence of AMI (22.1%) compared to adults aged 26-49 years (21.1%) and aged 50 and older (14.5%).
In 2016, there were an estimated 10.4 million adults aged 18 or older in the United States with SMI. This number represented 4.2% of all U.S. adults.

> The prevalence of SMI was higher among women (5.3%) than men (3.0%). Young adults aged 18-25 years had the highest prevalence of SMI (5.9%) compared to adults aged 26-49 years (5.3%) and aged 50 and older (2.7%). (NIMH, 2020)

The darkest side of mental health issues lies with the negative end results. Suicide is the tenth leading cause of death in the United States, accounting for about 47,000 people each year (SAMHSA, 2017). Rising rates of suicide are driving a shocking increase in the death rate of working-age Americans. Almost seventy-five percent of people with mental disorders remain untreated in developing countries with almost one million people taking their lives each year. In addition, according to the World Health Organization (WHO), one in thirteen, globally, suffer from anxiety.

Currently the effectiveness of antidepressants is between eleven and thirteen percent (Ioannidis, 2008). I bet most people are not aware of that. New research is showing that mental illness is a brain problem that can be managed through strengthening the brain and creating better neural networks, so maybe it is time to leave the ineffective drugs behind and find a real solution. As was the case with me, the pain medications and muscle relaxers may have taken away the pain I was feeling and the tightness in the chest, but at the same time, my spinal cord was being choked out and I was developing paralysis. If they had found the root cause of my symptoms, who knows whether they could have stopped it from happening—or at least mitigated it? Treatment has to be more about treating the patient and finding the root cause, instead of just fighting the symptoms and trying to quiet them. Again, in my case, it was the adjustment that woke up my brain and allowed me to feel pain and temperature again. No drug that had been tried on me up to that point had any positive effect.

It has been well-documented and reported lately that the drugs most often prescribed for ADHD can cause things like psychosis and other severe neuropsychological disorders. There has to be a better option for people who suffer with that condition.

Let's say you want to skip the pills and try a different solution. Well, if you go to a functional medicine doctor, they will do lab tests and look into a metabolic or dietary cause of your problems. This will likely result in supplements or dietary changes to affect your physiology and metabolism. If you go to a psychologist, then they will likely educate you on the emotional implications of your neurological disease. They may use talk therapy, or other methods like NeuroEmotional Technique, EMDR, or brainspotting. Other health care professionals may tell you that you need to move more and exercise.

I think that all of these explanations have merit in some way. They all tell part of the story. In chiropractic, we are trained with a vitalist mindset and taught about something referred to as subluxation, which is most simply understood as an interference in the nervous system. I will break down the nervous system in a minute, but in general, we are taught that there are three causes of interference: trauma, thoughts, and toxins.

From that point of view, all these conditions result from an interference in the nervous system, so all current theories that seek to explain the rise in these conditions have some merit and probably play a part in the root cause of what ails us.

We are going to take a look at how traumas, thoughts, and toxins affect the nervous system and what that means to your overall health. We are also going to learn what can be done about it without the use of drugs or surgery. I am not saying that drugs, surgery, or the doctors who utilize them for treatment are inherently bad—I just believe that there are natural cures out there that should be utilized first in our pursuit of health and well-being. When given the chance, they can actually be very effective without any of the negative consequences drugs and surgery can bring.

What's in a name? A rose by any other name smells as sweet. What's in a diagnosis?

Sometimes a diagnosis is just a Latin name that describes your symptoms. Sometimes the patient tells the doctor what the diagnosis is when they walk in. Other times a diagnosis may be a collection of symptoms that fit together, supported by a blood test or imaging study.

The problem with both blood tests and imaging studies is that even though they are currently the best way for us to look inside your body, they don't always say what we think they say. For instance, we think that if you have a disk bulge in your lower back (meaning one of the little shock absorbers that you have in your spine is broken) this will lead to back pain, but in a study published in the American Journal of Neuroradiology in December 2015, they found that many times a disk bulge was an incidental finding in people who didn't report symptoms of pain at all.

So, wait—if you have a disk bulge but no pain, does that mean it is the disk bulge that is a problem or not? If you have a bulge and no pain, there is no diagnosis for this. Really, what are we diagnosing when we call a disk bulge with pain "radiculopathy?" We are again just diagnosing symptoms.

Think about that. Most diagnoses are a collection of symptoms that you told your doctor you had, or that come from a test that could have been an incidental finding. So, is the name of your condition really anything, or could it just be a name that the doctor calls you?

In many cases, a diagnosis is just a word that describes the symptoms we told to the doctor, yet it can be very damaging to the person who receives the diagnosis. It is important for people to understand that a diagnosis is just an opinion. It is not a prison sentence or a branding. It is not who you are or who you have to become.

Too often, people start to become their diagnosis and lose all hope of ever regaining their former life. That is why I struggle with assigning a diagnosis to a case; I believe that the minute you give it a name, it begins to limit that person's outlook of their condition and expectation for their future.

Now don't get me wrong—I understand that there are conditions. When a person gets a diagnosis for a condition, it opens doors for them to receive help with support that they may not have had available to them without that diagnosis. However, we still need to look at the diagnosis differently.

A diagnosis is not a death sentence or a limitation, but a challenge to our minds to see if we can overcome this obstacle that has been placed in front of us. Can you climb the mountain that is in your way? Can you help your child or yourself get through this? Can we rise above what they tell us we can't do?

The mind and our thoughts shape our DNA. Our minds control every cell in our body. If we can move our thoughts past the limits of the "name" of our disease, what is really possible for us to overcome? I hope that these stories will inspire someone to look past the obstacles that have been placed before them to overcome and thrive in life.

Hans Selye, credited with unlocking our understanding of stress and our bodies' physiological responses to stress, was one the most brilliant medical minds of the past. One of his famous quotes reads, "Adapting the right attitude can convert a negative stress into a positive one." In other words, this can mean taking that negative event in your life and using it to fuel your drive to make a difference in the world. This stress or diagnosis or negative opinion of your health can be the catalyst to change your life for the better and unlock your true potential, or it can enslave you to a limited life of suffering. The choice is yours.

Even in blood tests or genetic testing we can only give patients a probability that they will develop a certain disease. That means that even if you have the genetic markers or a high or low lab value for something, it isn't written in stone that you *will* develop that something.

Again, don't get me wrong—if your blood sugar is high and you do not make changes, it will cause a disease process and you can die, but research says that with proper, informed lifestyle choices you can and will avoid those conditions. The blood and genetic markers, which we often assumed were a death sentence, are modifiable with lifestyle changes. The very ones that we supposedly don't control and supposedly can't do anything about.

Even with those markers we can only give you a probability. The difference in the people who don't develop the condition is that they did not limit themselves with the thought of the disease.

I know I am kind of trashing the idea that we need to diagnose. I don't mean to come off that way. We do need to have a way to classify conditions and to get people to the right person to care for them. I just want to introduce a new thought process of how we look at diagnoses as both a patient and as a doctor. What might be more appropriate is if we looked for the physiological cause of the condition. Meaning, instead of the question, "How are you feeling?" we should ask, "What made you feel this way?"

With that question, the answers can be wide-open. With that question, the solution to symptoms won't always just be a pill. With that question, there wouldn't be nearly as many limitations when it comes to breakthroughs in health and science.

—— CHAPTER THIRTEEN ——

THE NEW SCIENCES

We can always transcend and push barriers. At the time of my writing this book, just a few weeks ago someone ran a marathon in under two hours, something previously thought to be impossible. Just like the four-minute mile years ago, the two-hour marathon will quickly become the standard. We may never have to accept a new normal, so long as we don't accept limitations.

We are surrounded by wonderful technologies that give us the ability to know in real time what is going on in our systems. New insights into how our brain and body work together—and even how our soul plays into things—are exploding every day. As technology allows us to measure things more accurately and finely, we have gained new insights and even created some new sciences along the way. These sciences may help to unlock how we can heal from things that, in the past, were considered death sentences. We can now break through limitations that were once put on our minds' and bodies' abilities to heal. What some of these sciences are starting to show is that *there are no limitations.*

Vitalism

The definition of vitalism from Merriam-Webster Dictionary states, "a doctrine that the functions of a living organism are due to a vital principle distinct from physiochemical forces," or "that the processes of life are not explicable by the laws of physics and chemistry alone and that life is in some part self-determining" (Vitalim n.d.). Vitalism explicitly invokes a vital principle, which some equate with the soul. In the eighteenth and nineteenth centuries, vitalism was discussed among biologists, between those who felt that the known mechanics of physics would eventually explain the difference between life and nonlife, and vitalists, who argued that the processes of life could not be reduced to a mechanistic process. Some vitalist biologists proposed testable hypotheses meant to show inadequacies with mechanistic explanations, but these experiments failed to provide support for vitalism.

Elizabeth Ann Williams was a renowned author and biologist in the 1740s when these experiments were being run. In their research, they denounced the ideas of vitalism and dismissed them from medicine. Because of Williams's book, *A Cultural History of Medical Vitalism in Enlightenment,* from the eighteenth century, many biologists still refute the idea of vitalism. Biologists now consider vitalism, in this sense, to have been refuted by empirical evidence, and hence regard it as a superseded scientific theory (Dracobly, 2004).

Traditional health care has dismissed vitalism, saying that it was disproved because of an experiment run in the early part of the eighteenth century that showed the creation of an organic compound. Organic compounds are made from carbon and, at that point, had been thought could only come from living organisms. That theory was disproved by Friedrich Wöhler, in 1828, when he showed that heating silver cyanate (an inorganic, or nonliving, compound) with ammonium chloride (another inorganic compound) produced urea (an organic compound) without the aid of a living organism (Britannica, 2020). What this meant was that if they could create organic material in a lab, there could not be some unknown substance to life or soul.

This is great chemistry, but it is just that. Chemistry. When we look at vitalism through just a chemistry lens, it looks like the proof needed to disprove the theory—but even using that lens is flawed.

Those scientists tried to separate living and nonliving entities by a classification of organic versus inorganic compounds. That is to say, living tissue is organic (made from carbon) and nonliving tissue is inorganic (not made from carbon). But even this is currently debated, since there is not a consensus on what "counts" as living versus nonliving. This debate can be pretty intense, from looking into whether or not stem cells should be used, to debating whether or not something ceases to be "living" if it is picked from the tree from which it grew. Essentially this debate has become about determining when life begins and ends and how we play a part in that.

In addition, advances in science and the advent of new branches of science—like quantum physics and epigenetics—have reopened the case on something that was supposedly solved. Even acupuncture, a discipline that has been around for over five thousand years, doesn't agree with this chemistry thought process. With our new understanding (and admittedly, still incomplete knowledge) we are able to take this to the next level.

Quantum Physics and Our Understanding of the Universe

Everyone gets intimidated when you mention quantum physics. You don't even need the word "quantum" in front of "physics" to intimidate most. I am by no means an expert in this field, however, at this point you really need at least a basic understanding in some of the concepts to be in neuroscience (and, in my opinion, health care in general).

The term *quantum* applies to "an amount of something." When we put it into the name "quantum physics," this means "a discrete quantity of energy proportional in magnitude to the frequency of the radiation it represents." Or, in simpler terms, quantum physics is "the study of energy and how it interacts with the world." Where this gets a little dicey is when we describe human beings as energy. This is where our current understanding is headed, though, and in many health care disciplines we're already there.

In this book we are definitely not going into the really complex theories, but I want to touch on the idea of looking at things as photons. "Photons" is just a fancy way of saying "light," really, or "the particles that make up light."

Human beings are technically classified as matter, which isn't energy—but it also isn't *not* energy, if you are still with me. Matter is the hard substance and energy is the substance that animates and gives life to the matter. So, maybe we are matter, but we are *also* energy.

Since we know light is energy, and *we* are also partially energy, we can be partially described in the same way as we describe light. When we understand that we are made up of matter but that we are also made up of (and act like) photons, we can open our minds to the possibilities of quantum physics and how it affects us. It is possible to do this in a number of ways. Meditation is just one of them.

When we start looking at our physiological processes and how our body works, it is much better summed up in terms of energy and light than it is in terms of matter. Chemistry, after all, deals mostly with the physical world, where physics is more the science of energy.

To look at ourselves as energy and to talk in those terms, we need to use different vocabulary—musical terms, like tone, frequency, amplitude, wavelength, and depth.

> tone
> /tōn/
> noun
> 1.
> a musical or vocal sound with reference to its pitch, quality, and strength.
> "the piano tone appears monochrome or lacking in warmth"
> 2.
> the general character or attitude of a place, piece of writing, situation, etc.
> "my friend and I lowered the tone with our oafish ways"
>
> verb
> 1.
> give greater strength or firmness to (the body or a part of it).
> "exercise tones up the muscles"
> 2.
> harmonize with (something) in terms of color.

"the rich orange color of the wood tones beautifully with the yellow roses" (Tone, 2020).

Tone is simply the overall attitude of a situation. In music, it refers to the overall sound or "feel" of a piece. In the human body, it refers to muscle tone—muscle definition and a firm body indicates good "tone" in the muscles, or a positive, overall attitude of the muscles. In my world, a well-"toned" body means the nerves are flowing freely and keeping the muscle tight with constant information.

There isn't much difference from how we use this term with neuroscience. When we think of the tone of the brain and nervous system, we think of it in terms of regular flow from the brain to the body and back. We want good, appropriate flow with good control of the whole system—muscles as well as the immune, endocrine, digestive, cardiovascular, and other systems.

Believe it or not, your overall attitude is a good indicator of your current "tone," in terms of neuroscience. Someone who has a good, happy demeanor is indicative of someone with a strong brain and good health. A person with a poor attitude who struggles with depression or anxiety is a sign of poor tone of the nervous system and can indicate a weakness in the brain. D.D. Palmer, the father of chiropractic, used this term early on when describing the health of an individual. He was ahead of his time in this respect. In neuroscience, they use the similar term *the central integrated state* to refer to the activity in the nerves and parts of the nervous system. We can measure this central integrated state with technology like EEG.

Palmer was describing something over a hundred years ago that we have just now become able to measure. Think about how we will look back in the next hundred years. What will we be able to measure tomorrow that is only theory, today?

frequency
fre·quen·cy
/ˈfrēkwənsē/
noun
1.
the rate at which something occurs or is
repeated over a particular period of time or in
a given sample.
"shops have closed with increasing frequency
during the period"
2.
the rate at which a vibration occurs that con-
stitutes a wave, either in a material (as in sound
waves), or in an electromagnetic field (as in
radio waves and light), usually measured per
second (Frequency, 2020).

Frequency, when it comes to vibrations, refers to oscilla-
tions per second and is measured in hertz. Frequency is where
the information, or the knowledge, is stored—the frequency is
the meat of the thing. When we look at brain maps, a new technology that has unlocked a vast understanding of the brain, we
talk in terms of how the brain communicates with different frequencies. For instance, a beta wave or a delta wave may be carrying information that tells the brain how to better understand
its environment and how to best react to it.

Simply, the cells in the brain communicate information to
each other through waves that vibrate at various frequencies;
the faster the wave, the higher hertz (Hz) number associated
with it. For instance, a beta frequency might be 12 Hz, or have
a speed of twelve. That frequency is associated with an activity,
and in this case one cell is saying to another, "Get up and get

going." A delta wave, in contrast, might only be 2 Hz. That is like one cell saying to the other, "Hey take a nap and calm down. Let's just chill."

You should have all waveforms present in different areas of the brain at different times, but how much and at what time can give insight into brain problems or dysfunctions. We have even gotten to the point where we have databases of specific brain issues, like ADHD or a concussion, so we know what a common brain wave pattern looks like in that condition versus in a healthy brain.

A delta wave should be present in the brain in its highest concentrations when we are sleeping. Delta waves are made in the brain stem and then wash over the brain to create sleep. This wave is a message sent by special cells that give the orders to other cells to relax and rest so they can regenerate.

A beta wave should occur when our brain is active. These beta waves are generated by the front part of our brain, the frontal lobes, and this is a message of activity coming from these cells to drive other cells. Dr. Joe Dispenza, renowned neuroscientist, researcher, and author, has shown the presence of alpha, theta, and gamma waves during meditation and done research on how these different frequencies, when tapped into properly, can unlock the healing potential of the human brain, body, and spirit. Other people like Dr. Patrick Porter, a psychologist who studied at the University of Michigan, have developed technologies with binaural beats and isochronic tones to put your brain into certain brain waves almost on command. Technologies like this can vastly improve one's sleep, stress, anxiety, and so on.

We are really only beginning to scratch the surface on the implications that certain frequencies can have on health. Even the colors we look at have specific frequencies. For instance, red, depending on the shade, might be 396 Hz and green might be 528 Hz. When that frequency is perceived by the receptors in your eyes, you see color. But that same frequency also has a sound. So, you could effectively be looking at 528 Hz *and* listening to it at the same time. Michael Tyrell's Wholetones system has begun to marry the sound and visual of frequency to further unlock the potential of the brain. We already know that the brain and nervous system communicate in different frequencies—imagine what more we can unlock about the brain when we figure out how to better communicate with it using its language. These simple properties of sounds, colors, and waves could result in remarkably effective treatment someday.

am·pli·tude
/ˈamplə̩t(y)o͞od/
noun
noun: amplitude; plural noun: amplitudes
1.
PHYSICS
The maximum extent of a vibration or oscillation measured from the position of equilibrium.
the maximum difference of an alternating electrical current or potential from the average value.
2.
ASTRONOMY
the angular distance of a celestial object from the true east or west point of the horizon at rising or setting.

3.
breadth, range, or magnitude.
"the amplitude of the crime of manslaughter
lies beneath murder" (Amplitude, 2020).

Amplitude, in the body or nervous system, is best understood by thinking about intensity. When we work with patients who have certain conditions, like multiple sclerosis, Lyme disease, or seizures, they may be pretty sensitive. When working with someone who cannot handle a lot of stimulation, we have to be really careful to use activities with a low amplitude so we do not over activate their brain.

We want to feed their brain with activity to help it to heal, but if we give too much, we can crash the system—like if your house were to get a power surge. A little power running through your electrical wires and electrical system keeps the house running and the lights on. However, too much too quickly can create a surge and blow out light bulbs or your television. Well, your brain doesn't have the ability to use a power strip or surge protector, so we have to be careful how much activity we give the brain, especially when working with the brain of someone who is a little more sensitive. That is why, in some cases, we have to work very slowly—and so does the person's brain.

wave·length
/ˈwāv‚leNG(k)TH/
noun
1.
PHYSICS
the distance between successive crests of a wave, especially points in a sound wave or electromagnetic wave.

2.
a person's ideas and way of thinking, especially as it affects their ability to communicate with others.
"when we met, we hit it off immediately—we're on the same wavelength" (Wavelength, 2020).

Wavelength, in the brain, is best understood as language of the activity. You may remember a quote, usually done in a hippie voice, saying, "You just aren't on my wavelength, *man*." This means that you aren't using the same idea or language. Two people in a room talking to each other who are not using the same language results in nothing getting understood. This can happen in neurotherapy, sometimes. We have a patient who needs help learning to balance. A tool that we often use for balance training is a vibration plate, a plate that vibrates at different frequencies to activate the brain. However, some patients really cannot handle this, and it will throw them off. As soon as the plate gets turned on, they can fall over. We know that they need to better understand where their feet are in order to have better balance, but that signal wasn't on their wavelength so it confused them, and they fell over. A different signal, like a chiropractic adjustment or light touch, may be more appropriate for their system.

depth
/depTH/
noun
noun: depth; plural noun: depths; plural noun: the depths
1.
the distance from the top or surface to the bottom of something...

2.

the quality of being intense or extreme…

3.

a point far below the surface…

"a remote little village somewhere in the depths of Russia" Depth (Depth, 2020).

Depth is a little more abstract, as it relates to how your brain is turned on. However abstract, this term is very important for us humans. Depth refers to the richness of the experience. It can be thought of as the number of different receptors involved in an experience. This can be really huge for our brains. Think of this example: if you see a postcard of a really pretty landscape, like the forest or the beach, the picture will activate a lot of areas of your brain. You will get a good feeling and probably even relive a positive memory from that place or a place like it. You will remember a smell or a sound, and that area of your brain that perceives smell or sound will activate a little bit.

However, the depth of the experience will not equal the depth of actually being there. Actually smelling the smells and hearing the sounds will activate your brain on a much deeper level and much more profoundly than simply seeing the picture. Actually being there activates the brain many times more.

I often use the example of a digital encounter with a "friend" versus actually meeting up with that person in real life. There is a much deeper connection in real life, and thus deeper brain activation in person-to-person contact. That is why having personal relationships is so important to brain health. No amount of Facebook friends can change that.

Epigenetics

In October of 1990, an international scientific project was begun called the Human Genome Project (HGP). The project's goal was to determine the base pairs that make up human DNA, and to identify and map the human genome from both a physical and a functional standpoint. Simply put, the intent of this project was to unlock the basic building blocks of human DNA to determine how they performed and gave us the traits that make us, "us," from the color of our eyes to our chances of developing heart disease. The hope of this project was to give us better insight into helping prevent and treat the diseases that plague mankind.

However, there were unseen limits to this project. They were successfully able to map the human genome and determine the base pairs that make up DNA, but what they didn't understand at the time was how those genes came to be expressed. Genes tell only a portion of the story. While they do help to determine functional traits like eye color, hair color, and even body type, there were limits in accurately determining the risks of diseases.

For instance, two siblings may both be born with the same genetic predisposition to develop breast cancer. This means the two people will have the same risk when they are born to get the gene for breast cancer, but it doesn't mean they will both actually develop breast cancer. With genetics, we get some genes from Mom and some from Dad. If one parent has the gene for cancer and the other does not, the child has between a twenty-five and fifty percent chance of getting the gene for cancer.

All that is old genetic science. The interesting part that we have seen lately in science is that even if you have the gene for cancer, you don't always develop that cancer, or any other disease you may have the genes for. This brought up the question of what determines whether or not you present that gene and develop what the gene codes for.

This brings up the age-old biological and psychological debate of nature versus nurture. If you think back, you may remember this argument from high school biology and psychology classes. Which, nature or nurture, has a greater influence over who we become? Is it more about the genes that make up our body, or the environment we grow up in? Even after the completion of the Human Genome Project, that debate still wages on.

The reality is that it is probably a bit of both. The new science supports that the genes passed down to us from our parents are a big player in how we develop, but it might be the environment that gets the last laugh, so to speak, since the environment can affect the genes that you have and mold which genes get expressed or suppressed. You have genes for multiple things, and sometimes you even have two opposite pairs of genes. The environment that they are put in can determine which gene pair gets expressed. For example, you could have a gene that increases your risk for heart disease and a gene that allows for proper functioning of the heart, and the foods you eat, the air you breathe, or even how you handle stress in your life can change which gene gets to be expressed.

In the past, people have thought about it in terms of a gene "turning on or off." Certain activities or environments were thought to turn on the gene for heart disease and certain environments turn off that gene. For instance, always eating a lot of fats and sugars will turn on the genes that develop type 2 diabetes or certain cancers. Rather than a light switch, the more appropriate way to think about it is the gene being *expressed* or *suppressed*. The difference being, our DNA doesn't get turned off or on. Your DNA is simply the determining factor in what products your cells make. Under certain circumstances, they can create good, useful, functional products, but under other circumstances, they can create dysfunctional products.

I grew up in Michigan around the Big Three—that is, Ford, Chrysler, and General Motors. They were the pride of the Midwest in the earlier part of the twentieth century. However, the workers were overworked and underpaid, and fatigue and low morale caused a decrease in the quality of the product that they were producing. In May of 1935, the Auto Workers Union was created to help protect the autoworkers from inhumane working conditions. This change in the environment created a happier, healthier workspace, and in turn created a better product. Our bodies are no different. When they have the proper building blocks and are breathing good air with good fuel, they create a healthier environment. The idea of our genes being able to express differently isn't really a new idea. It has just begun to build popularity lately.

The idea that genes can change their expression is known as epigenetics. *Epigenetics* was first coined in 1942 by a British embryologist named Conrad H. Waddington, who used the term to talk about the changes that happened in an egg during fertilization. Over the next fifty years the term evolved, but let's take this example to explain how something can change the way it functions based on environmental changes. When an egg is fertilized, the products created by the cells change. It receives different chemical and energetic signals. These changes in signals tell the cell that it needs to change its response to the environment. In the case of a fertilized egg, the job is no longer to just protect and carry the DNA signature of the mother but to now begin the creation of life, and so the cell starts to create different things like proteins to carry out that new job.

Our bodies, nervous systems, and cells are encoded with a need to survive and carry on the human race. You will hear this theme over and over as we explain some case studies in this book. In order to survive, our cells will give up all sorts of comforts they deem unnecessary. Our cells will change the way that they respond to the environment based on what stressors or threats are out there.

A scientist by the name of Bruce Lipton is one of the most recent researchers to really bring the idea of epigenetics back to the forefront. In his book, *The Biology of Belief,* he outlines the cell processes that he researched in his lab. The DNA in our cells is the blueprint for the creation of the products of the cell, but DNA isn't the be-all and end-all. The DNA blueprint is influenced by the outside environment. Your DNA is altered by the air you breathe, the food you eat, and even the thoughts that you think. DNA is a blueprint to tell your cells what proteins need to be made to do the job of the cell. If you change your environment, you will change the job of the cell. This means that you can have DNA for a few different jobs. The environment you are in will determine which one needs to be done, and the cell will use that part of the DNA to get that job done.

Another key aspect of this thought process Dr. Lipton introduces is that this environment is not only the air we breathe and food that we eat, but also our thoughts—both negative and positive. Think about that. We actually have some control over the environment in our bodies that changes the way our DNA responds to the universe.

MIND = BLOWN!

This is because your body will respond to and get good at what you tell it to do. If you have negative thoughts all the time, the pathways in your brain for fear, anxiety, and preparing for the worst will be activated more than the ones for seeing the big picture and experiencing happiness and joy. When this happens, the cells in the "fear" parts of the brain become more active and then require more energy. When those cells require more energy, they require the cell to make more proteins and substances to carry out their job. So, the DNA and chromosomes that help with those specific proteins get expressed more often and eventually become the default. If this happens, other proteins for other parts of the brain (for happiness and joy) will get suppressed or "turned off." Then the pathways for those emotions will become harder to trace—and those emotions will become harder to feel. As a result of these changes, your physiology changes and you produce different chemicals that are set up more around stress. Then stress becomes your new set point. If stress is your body's "comfortable" default, it will react with stress to everything. This is how your body becomes acidic and can start to deteriorate your system. The same proteins that are created for fear and anxiety cause your system to become more acidic.

When he first introduced these ideas, it was considered to be pretty "out-there" science. However, with today's advances in psychology, quantum physics, and neuroscience, we have begun to support some of the previously "out-there" sciences. We are really just beginning to understand *how* the body interacts with its environment, but we do know our thoughts and beliefs *can* affect our physiology and the inner workings of our bodies. Really, the theories about this are not as new as we may think. Before Dr. Lipton showed that our thoughts affect our DNA, Dr. Hans Selye was showing that thoughts affect our physiology as well, causing our cells to break down, leading to disease.

Hans Selye was a medical doctor in the late 1930s who first began to notice similarities in many disease processes he saw. While in medical school, his professors would parade all the different pathologies in front of the class to show the clinical signs and symptoms unique to each condition, but Selye saw something else. Where others were feverishly writing down the hallmarks of such conditions as diabetes, cancer, and heart disease, Selye was noting the similarities, and beginning to understand a common thread that connected all of these conditions.

That thread was that the cells in these patients had lost the ability to adapt to the environment that they were in. The stressors in their world were beginning to break down cell processes. To put it in epigenetics terms, the patient's stress was forcing the body's cells to create different products and express different genes in an attempt to survive. Unfortunately, sometimes what the cells and body believe is best ends up being a poor adaptation. Maybe it is the cells seeing the dysfunction and ending that program so that it doesn't carry on in the species, or maybe that adaptation is simply going to get the most days out of that organism. Either way, he saw that these adaptations were similar in many different conditions.

For instance, in all the chronic conditions that they brought before the class—like diabetes, cancer, and chronic pain—the patients showed elevated heart rate, elevated blood pressure, fatigue, and mood changes. This was the response of the body to help fight the condition; it had to pull resources from the areas of the brain and body that helped to regulate these things. Dr. Selye gave us the framework to understand our stress responses and figure out how outside influences, even mental ones, were influencing the physiology and function of our bodies at a cellular level. In addition to the obvious physiological markers like blood pressure and heart rate, Dr. Selye also noticed that these patients had aspects of depression, anxiety, and other poor mental and emotional responses to the conditions.

One of my favorites, Hunter Doherty Adams, saw this in practice too. You might know him as Patch Adams from the eponymous movie. Yes, the man Robin Williams so brilliantly portrayed was an actual physician. In fact, when you look at his biography on patchadams.org, he is listed as an American physician, comedian, social activist, clown, and author. He realized that a large part of healing was having hope and a positive mindset. He believed that in order to get your body and cells to heal and regenerate, you first needed to get your head right. He founded the Gesundheit! Institute in 1971. Taken from his website, patchadams.org:

The Gesundheit Institute was a pilot hospital model, which we operated for twelve years out of our communal home. We were always open for any kind of problem.

Our policy was:
1. no charge
2. no health insurance reimbursement
3. no malpractice insurance
4. three- to four-hour initial interview with the patient
5. home as hospital
6. integration of all the healing arts
7. integration of medicine with performance arts, arts and crafts, nature, agriculture, education, recreation and social service
8. the health of the staff is as important as the health of the patient.

We did this for twelve years and saw thousands of patients. The experience was enchanting (Gesundheit!, 2020).

Adams understood that people who are suffering need compassion, and above all need to be treated as a person. Even though the Gesundheit Institute failed to get enough funding to continue as planned, Adams continues to push on with global outreach events, bringing happiness to the sick all around the world.

Think about what our world would be like if all hospitals functioned like this!

When you combine this with the research by Waddington and then carried on by Lipton, you can see why this theory is gaining a deeper understanding and getting more support from the scientific and research communities.

Even though this science is still developing and is still in an early stage of its development, it is giving us a framework for a better understanding of some clinical changes we are seeing. Putting together some of the breakthroughs in biology with those of physics, psychology, and neurology is unlocking a deeper understanding of the human body. The idea that we are just a collection of chemical processes is starting to fade. The idea that we can have better health through chemistry alone is being challenged, as we see the failures of that thought process. We are beginning to understand that the human form is complex and bridges all of the sciences. We will need the coming together of all current branches of science (and more branches we haven't discovered yet) to really understand what's going on.

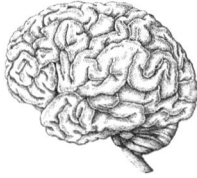

CHAPTER FOURTEEN

NEUROPLASTICITY AND MOVEMENT

Our brains and nervous systems are two of the most complex and important parts of who we are, and yet we still understand very little of how they work. Even though there are advances in our understanding of their inner workings almost daily, we still have so many questions. Neuroscience is constantly researching conditions such as Alzheimer's and Parkinson's, injuries such as concussion and stroke, and even the existence of consciousness and the difference between the mind and the brain in an attempt to answer some of our pressing questions.

One fairly recent discovery in neuroscience is the understanding of neuroplasticity. Neuroplasticity shows us that an old brain *can* learn new tricks—in other words, the brain can be reformatted or rewired. Areas can be repurposed to take over function for an area that has been damaged or that can no longer do its job so we can maintain function. This is a very important principle in our understanding of the brain. It offers insight into so many disorders of the brain and nervous system, but more importantly it also shows us the way to heal our most important organ.

Neuroplasticity was, until recently, very controversial. Even though Karl Lashley first proposed the idea of neuroplasticity in 1923, it wasn't until 1964 when Marian Diamond of the University of California, Berkeley, produced the first scientific evidence of anatomical brain plasticity. And it wasn't until 2016 that Michael Merzenich won the Nobel Prize for proving we retain the ability to make brain changes throughout our lifetime. Until his findings, it was thought that we only had neuroplasticity, or the ability to change the brain, early on in life. The assumption was that children had the ability to change their brains, but adults did not. However, Dr. Merzenich proved adults could also change their brains. I have seen neuroplastic changes in people as old as ninety-one, who were able to make lasting improvements in cognitive function—despite the onset of the early stages of dementia.

Epigenetics focuses on how the environment changes genetic expression. Neurology focuses on how the environment and information being received by the brain can change your neurological networks and function—otherwise known as neuroplasticity. The understanding of neuroplasticity has revolutionized neuroscience.

Even though the brain is a very complex organ, when you really think about it, it only has three jobs: perceive, process, and react. It just needs to be able to perceive our environment—or take in sensory signals, like sight, sound, smell, and touch—process that information, and then form a response to the information. The brain has a very intricate network of structures to do all this seemingly instantly. In fact, it happens so fast that some neuroscientists actually believe the brain only has two jobs: first to predict the future, and second to adjust if it is wrong. The complexity, and controversy, in this is *how* it actually gets these jobs done.

Another major job of the brain is in regulation or control. This is actually the number one job of what we picture when we picture the brain, the wrinkly part that has all the folds and ridges. This is the cortex part of the brain, and it is responsible for controlling all of the organs and cells in our bodies. It controls our emotions, heart rate, metabolism, temperature regulation, hunger, growth, and all other processes that our body and nervous system have to carry out. This is important because when the brain is damaged or not functioning at its best, this control is affected.

Many neurological diseases have symptoms of this lack of control, like poor focus or attention; poor control over emotions like anxiety, sadness, or anger; trouble controlling our sugar, such as with diabetes; and even trouble controlling our heart rate and blood pressure, like in hypertension. Sound familiar? These are all some very common disorders that many people in our society suffer with today, and all of those processes are regulated by your brain. Not to say that the brain is the only reason for these problems, but it *is* the master system. Diet and other lifestyle factors can affect these things as well.

Let's go back to the simplified version of the brain's responsibilities: perception, processing, and reacting. We know that there can be a breakdown in any one of these, and whichever system is breaking down will determine the presentation of symptoms and even how severe the case may be. But we also know that through the process of creating neuroplastic change, all these systems can be fixed or rewired. One way to do so is through the principles of neuroscience and the utilization of receptors to affect change in the brain. We call this receptor-based therapy.

Receptors are the parts of your nervous system that sense your environment. Receptors in our eyes, for instance, receive light and send those signals to the brain to interpret. If someone has an uncorrected vision problem, their visual input will not be appropriate; they will not be able to perceive distance correctly, they will process the incoming visual information incorrectly, and they will then react poorly. When they try to grab an object they're reaching for, they will reach past it and may even knock it over.

Receptors are all over the body—some perceive chemicals in the air or in food, which is how smell and taste work. Others are responsible for telling our brain where our body parts are in space, or for feeling pain, or for feeling things inside our organs. We can use and manipulate these receptors to change how the brain perceives the world around it and even its own body. If the perception changes, then so does the processing, and then, so will our response. If we get glasses, we won't knock things over anymore.

Negative thoughts can have a huge impact on how we perceive the world, process it, and react to it. They are also something we can affect that will result in a big change in our internal environment.

Perception controls behavior. Our behavior is our personality. Our personality determines our environment. Environment is perceived, and round and round it goes.

Traditionally, we think about behavior as attitude or personality. However, I want to introduce behavior as one of two things: our bodies can either be in a behavior of fight-or-flight, or in a behavior of rest-and-digest. These phases come from the sympathetic and parasympathetic nervous systems, which control how the body responds based on whether or not we perceive the environment as a threat or a friend. Depending on the system that is running the show, our cells are going to go either into a breakdown mode or a building mode. In a breakdown mode, known as catabolism, cells break down to get used as energy to continue either fighting or fleeing the scene. In building mode, or anabolism, the cells think they are in an environment where it is safe to regenerate. This means that, since they don't have to use energy to run or fight, they go check if anything needs to be fixed and address whatever needs help.

If our sympathetic nervous system is running the show, our body and cells are perceiving the environment as threatening. When this occurs, our body gets really efficient at staying alive. This means it reverts resources like blood, oxygen, and energy to the areas of the brain, nervous system, and body that are responsible for staying alive.

Do you see how this could become an issue, if we are injured or in the hospital and need to be in a regenerative state? Hospitals are scary enough—the way they are laid out, the sterility of them, the loud sounds and everyone moving around like they are in a hurry all the time make it a pretty intimidating environment. This intimidation can put us into fight-or-flight mode pretty quickly. This can be a problem, considering what probably landed us in there in the first place.

We need things in the hospital that can help put our minds and bodies at ease, so to speak. Someone to help us understand what is going on with us and to tell us that we will be alright. Without that interaction, we are left to feel as though we are in a dangerous situation, and this causes our brain and body to react as such.

When the brain feels like it is in danger, it sends resources to an area of the brain known as the limbic system. The limbic system is the emotional part of the brain and it is responsible for feeling fear at the sight of an attacker. It also feels happy at the sight of food or shelter, and sad when we have loss. While this part of our brain is essential to survive, if our brains feel like they are always in danger and are constantly sending its resources to the limbic system, we begin to be run by our emotions. This isn't good for anyone.

I think this is a big problem with our society. We live with constant, instant information with the news in the palm of our hand twenty-four hours a day, seven days a week. With the slant of the news being toward fear, negative stories, and what we are struggling with in the world, consuming the news almost always puts us into this sympathetic part of our nervous system.

The good news is that we come built in with a part of our brain that is responsible for turning off this limbic control: the frontal lobe. This is the front part of our brains and, in addition to shutting down our limbic responses, it is also responsible for things like posture, executive thinking, seeing the big picture, and knowing everything is going to be alright.

The frontal lobe is activated through signals from another part of the brain called the cerebellum. The cerebellum is most activated through upright, weight-bearing movement, like running or walking. Think about it: we are bipedal. We walk upright. This is different from most animals and has helped us develop a bigger and stronger frontal lobe through pathways coming in from the cerebellum. When we are not moving, we struggle to control our emotions because the frontal lobe struggles to stay active enough to control the brain. When we are not moving, we become more primitive or animalistic.

When in fight-or-flight mode, in addition to changing the flow of resources in the brain, we also do the same thing in the body. We shunt resources and blood to the extremities, away from the gut—moving resources to the areas responsible for fighting or running. We don't need to digest our food while doing either one of those acts (you won't win many fights or races with a hamburger and fries in your hands, although that would be fun to watch).

Again, I think this is what we are seeing in our society. We have more food allergies and sensitivities than we ever had. It feels like everyone is allergic to gluten these days. We are becoming allergic to the foods we eat, the air we breathe, and just about everything around us, in part because of the way our body is responding to the world. When we are in that sympathetic nervous system, that fight-or-flight, we are not ready to digest food. We don't produce the right amount of chemicals to break down food and to line our gut, so food actually does some damage to that system as it passes through us. This makes our system upset further and gets us ready to fight again—a never-ending cycle. This causes a whole host of conditions: from weight gain that contributes to the obesity epidemic, to depression and anxiety that contribute to the mental health epidemic, to cancer, and other conditions.

The system of the body that is responsible for fighting things like viruses or bacteria that might hurt us is known as the immune system. What happens when the immune system starts to think of the food we eat as an invader? Yep, you guessed it: it will start to attack the food. That reaction looks like a sensitivity or an allergy to food that used to nourish us. Our immune systems are trying to protect us, and when we are in that fight-or-flight mode and eating our foods, we are telling our systems, through thought, that what is coming is an enemy. This then builds that immune system up to attack all sorts of things, even our own bodies.

When the immune system attacks its own body, we call it an autoimmune disease—examples include multiple sclerosis, ALS, and lupus. Even diseases like traumatic brain injury, Alzheimer's, ADHD, and Parkinson's have aspects of immune dysregulation or autoimmunity.

If our world and all that we are bombarded with activates our sympathetic nervous system and puts us into alarm mode, what can be done to combat this? Well, as we said, the frontal lobe—specifically an area known as the prefrontal cortex—is responsible for seeing the big picture. This area of the brain allows us to rationalize everything we are going through and to cognitively understand that we can and will move past this. It is the area of the brain that connects to others and to something bigger than us. It is the area of the brain that separates us from the rest of the animals in the animal kingdom. It gives us our ability to wait and hold back until an appropriate time.

When I speak to groups about neurology, I often use the example of the frontal lobe allowing us to wait until it is socially appropriate to act. In children, this area is not yet mature, which is why a three-year-old might climb on the counter to get a cookie even though they were told no, whereas I might actually be able to show some restraint from getting a cookie (notice I said I *might* be able to. Cookies are one of my known weaknesses). This development of the frontal lobe separates us from the animals, not just for the ability to reason but for our ability to be social and wait for appropriate times. We are able to hold back on our urges or desires and even on things that are necessary for survival. We should be able to hold back from stealing food from a friend, to preserve social ties. The rest of the animal kingdom does not always show the ability to have that restraint. Restraint is, in essence, humanity. The area that gives us these abilities is the prefrontal cortex, which gets its activation and energy from movement.

Movement is life.

In addition to the prefrontal cortex, the other area of the brain that relies on movement and is hugely implicated in control of our emotions and thoughts is the cerebellum. This area of the brain does not take up a lot of real estate inside the skull, but it has more neurons (brain cells) and makes more connections than the whole rest of the brain combined. In fact, the cerebellum only makes up ten percent of the total brain volume, even though it outnumbers the entire rest of the brain by ten to twenty-six *billion* in number of cells.

As recently as 2018, we didn't have a great understanding of this part of the brain. When I was in school, we were taught that all the cerebellum controlled was balance and coordination. However, recent science has begun to help us understand that we were ignorant in our understanding of this part of the brain. New research in 2018, brought to light because of new technology that could actually map the cerebellum, showed that the cerebellum was actually a major player in everything from our cognitive function (how well we learn) to our emotional regulation. It even has networks associated with controlling our immune function and balancing the sympathetic and parasympathetic networks. This gives a new importance and greater meaning to the idea that the cerebellum is in charge of "balance." What we see in our clinic is that good physical balance and movement usually equals good emotional balance as well, and vice versa.

The cerebellum (balance and coordination) and the frontal lobe (big picture and humanity) get activated most through upright, weight-bearing movement. More specifically they are most turned on through running and walking long distances.

In the book *Brain Rules*, best-selling author John Medina shows research that supports the idea that we should walk upwards of twelve miles a day. There is a growing amount of evidence that exercise including upright movement is needed for proper brain development (Perez, 2019), can help us heal from things like traumatic brain injury (Sharma, 2020), fight off depression (Ignacio, 2019), decrease mental issues in young people (Pascoe, 2020), and even reverse the brain's aging process and early neurodegeneration (Horowitz, 2020). We often say in our office that health is an active process. We need to move to be healthy, and we need to move with others. The sense of belonging to something bigger than ourselves is paramount in the activation of the frontal lobe and the cerebellum, and so it is paramount in our health and well-being.

In our office, we rewire the brain away from pain and dysfunction mostly through movement-based exercises. Remember the receptors all over your body? All information your receptors pick up goes through a filter in your brain known as the thalamus. This filter, with the help of your brain, determines what is important to let through and be consciously aware of—but make no mistake, your brain still processes all of it.

The collection of all the information that these little receptors send to your brain are making up what Dr. Michael Hall, Developer of BrainDC, would refer to it as "your reality." The signals that come in from your receptors are "sensory signals," and they form the basis for perception. Now, you also overlay all of that information with your past memories, too, which is why everyone perceives the world just a little bit differently—but more on that later. Your little receptors all take in a different part of the environment, and together give your brain a complete picture of what is going on around you.

Once our brain believes that it has the appropriate picture of its reality, it can form a movement, thought, or emotion about it. That is what Dr. Hall would call "your personality" (we believe it is much more complex than this, but for the purposes of this book, this is a good understanding). If you want to go a little further, as Dr. Joe Dispenza explains in his book, *Breaking the Habit of Being Yourself,* if we get enough of these reactions to the environment, we end up with our mood, and if we are in a mood for long enough, it becomes our demeanor, which eventually becomes just who we are.

Therefore, we really are just a collection of our perceptions of the world around us and how we react to them. But what if there is a breakdown in one of those channels of perception? What if the body doesn't get the most complete or accurate picture of the world around it? Do you think that will affect our reaction to it? The science says yes. If there is a breakdown in the way we are perceiving things, or even if we have a bad memory about something from our past, it will change our reaction to it and even change our body chemistry or physiology in reaction to it.

Think of it like this: if I were to hear the song "Everything About You" by Ugly Kid Joe, I get a little smile on my face because I think it is kind of a funny song. But if someone broke up with you while that song was playing, you would have a completely different physiological experience to hearing the same song. You might get flushed or angry, or even get a little queasy. The receptors were activated the same way with the same frequency in my ear and your ear. So why was our response so different? Memories. We each had a different association to that song, so our body responded to how it remembered it did before.

We don't just do that with music; we do that constantly with everything we are taking in. Isn't the brain amazing? We overlay our past experiences on everything that our receptors are taking in, so no two people ever truly experience the world in the same way. That is pretty crazy, if you really stop and think about it. For instance, when I see a wheelchair, I get a quick sinking feeling in the pit of my stomach. My association with the wheelchair is tied to anger, to someone telling me I would be confined to it with no other choice. However, someone else may look at a wheelchair and have happy memories if it reminded them of a loved one, like a grandparent, who was in a wheelchair at one point in their life.

The other crazy thing to think about is that those receptors are always on. They are always perceiving the environment we are in. For instance, right now the receptors for touch are active in your butt and in your feet. Until you read "butt" and "feet" you didn't feel yours, but now that you have read those words you are conscious of them. The receptors didn't just "turn on" when you read those words. They were always taking in the environment. But when you read "butt" and "feet" your brain stopped and said, "Wait, 'butt and feet,' that reminds me. I better check in with them and make sure they are alright."

The brain fired down to the thalamus, the filter, and said, "Let through information about the butt and the feet." Your brain made that information conscious so your higher centers could see what was going on.

Feel free to get up and stretch if you feel you just realized your butt is asleep or foot is cramping from sitting too long.

The thalamus is the gatekeeper of information. It only allows in who is on the guest list, and the guest list is determined by who the brain wants to check on. The brain then takes the information from the receptors and combines with its memories of related moments to determine what it is going on and whether or not it is truly important enough to act on. The information about the butt is either understood to be pain (and so we will move to get away from that painful stimulus) or it is determined unimportant, so you continue to sit and read. After a while, you will forget about it—the thalamus will block out its information again, and your higher brain will focus on something else again. This is happening all over your body, all the time. This highlights the importance of movement and the constant experiencing of your environment. Your brain needs previous memories to compare incoming information to, and it needs to exercise this skill of perception to do it effectively.

Just like how our body has specialized receptors to perceive the environment, our brain has specialized areas to process that information. For instance, the occipital cortex in the back of the head is where we process vision, and sound is processed in the temporal cortex, which is right behind your ears. The cool part about all these areas is that their primary function is not *all* they do. They have other jobs, and when they combine with other networks, they can really get a lot of things done. What else is cool is that when one of these areas gets damaged or loses function (or maybe doesn't develop correctly in the first place), other areas can pick up that function and help out. We can teach other areas to take over and help out to restore function.

We can use our receptors to make neuroplastic changes in the brain to improve function for a whole bunch of conditions. One of the biggest ways we can do that is with movement. Movement is the biggest bang for our buck, so to speak, because you have the most receptors dedicated to it, contributing to the perception of the world. I use the original chiropractic story to explain this.

Patient zero, if you will, in chiropractic was a guy by the name of Harvey Lillard. Harvey was a janitor in the office building where D.D. Palmer, the father of chiropractic, was practicing his craft. Harvey had difficulty hearing; in fact, he was legally deaf. One day, D.D. Palmer adjusted him using a chiropractic adjustment. Now the documentation isn't exact about where he adjusted him, but after he was adjusted, he got up and realized he could hear again. When I was in school, I thought this story was amazing, but scientifically it didn't make a lot of sense as to what I was learning in my classes.

We were learning about how the bone rests on the nerve, and how the bone dampens the nerve's function. And when you adjust someone, that function is restored because the pressure was removed from the nerve. Heck, that is what my chiropractor told me when he was helping me. When I first started with him, he told me that in some cases the bones in the spine can get stuck and push on nerves. This pressure was the source of pain and dysfunction. For a long time that was the understanding behind how a chiropractic adjustment could help people. But I pored through the anatomy books and could not find any nerve that had anything to do with hearing that also went anywhere near the spine, let alone originated in the spine. There wasn't any magic nerve in the spine to help with hearing. So how did this story make sense? And furthermore, how could this explain my story? Were all the bones resting on all the nerves? That wasn't probable and really with my current understanding is not possible. So how then did the adjustment restore my perception of hot and cold and even pain?

It wasn't until sitting in Dr. Michael Hall's class that the story started to become clear. Dr. Hall used a term called "central integrated state," a fancy term that basically refers to the collection of signals coming into the brain. It is the hum of the brain, so to speak, or the brain's resting activated state. He went on to explain that the signals from the receptors for movement, sound, sight, and so on all contribute to the central integrated state of the brain.

Harvey had a segment in his spine that wasn't moving, so he didn't have as much information contributing to that hum as someone else would who had all the segments moving freely. Therefore, his perception of the environment had decreased. Harvey had lost his ability to perceive sound, but in others it may result in bad balance, heart issues, or a whole host of symptoms and conditions. The chiropractic adjustment put a huge sensory barrage of information into his system and improved his ability to perceive the environment better. For Harvey, since his hearing had been affected, it was his hearing that was perceived as the biggest change.

That movement and information, delivered very specifically to the area that was messing with the input, restored the signal and brought the hum of the brain up—or, as D.D. Palmer referred to it, the tone of the nervous system. Science today refers to it as the central integrated state.

That is how powerfully movement can activate our brains, in a unique way, to bring about better function.

Perception is based not only on physical sensations but also our previous experiences or memories. We don't just take things in through the receptors, but we also filter them through our past experiences. That is why a bunch of people in a room together can experience the same event differently. I had a teacher in high school that really challenged this thought process with us. Now before I tell this story, I want to preface it by saying that this would never happen in school today. But I was in high school before Columbine, and before school shootings were really a "thing." Also, I grew up in a small town where many of the students had hunting rifles in their cars at school. This is absolutely not meant to offend or make light of issues with guns or with guns in or around our schools.

My history teacher, my sophomore year, had set up a test with another student. As we sat in class, we had no idea what was coming. My friend Aaron was sitting in the class in front of me. We were told to pull out our books and begin reading the chapter. While we were reading quietly, Aaron started to talk to someone in front of him. Mr. Brown quickly scolded him. Aaron took offence to the teacher's words and chirped back. Mr. Brown instructed Aaron to follow him out into the hall. You could hear the argument from inside the class and many of the students' jaws were dropped and others were laughing at the exchange between the two of them in the hallway.

All of sudden we heard bangs that sounded like little explosions. Everyone was startled, then nothing. A few minutes passed, what felt like twenty minutes and Mr. Brown reentered the classroom with Aaron grinning behind him. Mr. Brown promptly told everyone to pull out a piece of paper and a pencil and very specifically write down exactly what had just happened. Everyone followed the instructions and feverishly wrote down the exact events that just took place.

He told us, "I want to know how many bangs you heard, what was said, who started it, etc."

When we were all ready, he asked us to read the accounts out loud. We made it through quite a few, but none of them were the same. Each of us in the room had different things to say. The people that knew Mr. Brown as a coach had sided with him and said that Aaron had acted poorly, and that Aaron fired shots at Mr. Brown. Aaron's friends had said that he was never talking, and Mr. Brown picked on him when he called him out. It was eye-opening, and my first understanding of how we each see the world differently and have a different filter with how we perceive the world.

Our brains do this with everything. From the people we see on a daily basis, to the events that happen around us, and even our little unconscious perceptions that occur. We enter the day with our own filter on the world. Our limbic system makes sure of it. If we have had a negative experience the night before or wake up on the wrong side of the bed, we can set our day up to have negative experiences all day long. But the opposite is also true; if we wake up ready to attack the day with an enthusiasm unknown to mankind, like Jim Harbaugh, we can create a positive experience and see things through a more positive filter. This more positive filter could help us to keep that sympathetic nervous system at bay a little.

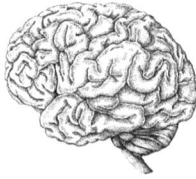

CHAPTER FIFTEEN

MOVEMENTS

Understanding that movements, thoughts, and emotions are processed by the same areas of the brain has been a breakthrough in cognitive and behavioral neuroscience.

Think about how movements can change the makeup of the body. Working out can exercise muscles and make them stronger and appear bigger. Well, emotions and thoughts can have the same effect on the pathways in the brain. We focus our energy and exercise our perceptions based on our thoughts and emotions. Just like an athlete can get very good at a specific action through practice, we can get really good at thinking a certain thought or feeling a certain emotion through practice. This is neuroplasticity at work.

However, neuroplasticity can be for the good or for the bad. If you keep thinking negative thoughts and emotions, then you will more easily stay in those negative thoughts and emotions.

Scientists have been studying for years now the effects that things like prayer, meditation, and positive thinking have on health—not just mental health, but also metabolic and physical health. One thing that is consistent with patients who suffer from any kind of sickness is that there is almost always an emotional or thought component.

We activate the brain by experiencing our environment through the receptors in our body. That activation feeds the brain with impulses and signals and allows us to wire pathways that control things like mood, heart rate, blood pressure, the immune system, and other reflexive systems in our body. If we regularly activate the brain with movement, we get the brain used to building muscle, prioritizing health, and feeling happy and accomplished.

When we don't move well or enough, we don't feed the frontal lobe of the brain or the cerebellum with activation. The movements and exercises that we know are necessary for keeping other structures in our body like the heart and lungs healthy also feed our brain. The system is set up for us to win. It is set up for us to move and be well.

When we don't move enough, we experience more fatigue, more sadness, and more depression. We also have a higher chance of developing other diseases like chronic pain, ADHD, Parkinson's, and Alzheimer's. Stress and a sedentary lifestyle can lead to the weakening of the brain and body.

In our office, we work with many complex neurological conditions, and there is an emotional component in every one of them. Now I don't mean that they were emotional or making it up, or that it was simply them "stressing out" about their health (even though that might be what was told to them by other doctors). It is actually quite the opposite. Most of our patients have had very obvious outward physical signs and symptoms of illness.

One patient was sixteen years old and had chronic pain at an eight out of ten throughout his body. His doctor, at a prestigious medical university, looked at his mother and said, "When your son wants to get better, he will be better. His only option at this point is a psychology referral."

Can you imagine being the mother of a sixteen-year-old, with a mission in life to make sure they are safe, and this doctor is telling you that everything you are trying to help them with is made up or all in his head?

Well, the doctors are right: it is all in your head, just not in the way that they think. Pain can, in fact, be all in your head, but that doesn't mean it isn't real. In my patient's brain, he had pain that had grown and gotten more intense over a short time. Well, just like learning a new skill, the brain interpreted this pain as something to learn. The longer the pain persisted, the more the brain wanted to get good at it because it thought that this was its new normal. So, by not finding a way to inhibit the pain early enough, the brain had been rewired to perceive pain, and it got really good at it—so good that medication and other traditional forms of treatment had no effect on it.

His pain had become hardwired so much on the left side of his body (the side the pain started on), that his body started to change its physiology. His body started to pull calcium out of his bones to help to deal with the perceived threat of pain. It pulled enough calcium out of his bones that when we did a bone scan on him, there was an eighteen percent decrease in both bone mineral composition and bone mineral density in *all* his bones on the left side of the body.

But it was all in his head, right? Well it was—his head, or brain, had become so wired for pain it started to change his internal environment or physiology. Even though he had this condition for so long it was changing his bones, his brain was still able to regain a healthier pattern and be trained out of his pain.

His brain became good at pain. We had to give it something else to get good at that was actually beneficial. We were able to activate the parts of his brain that were usually busy perceiving pain with other jobs. For instance, we gave the parietal lobe, the area of the brain that perceives touch, something else to feel. We had him focus on feeling vibrations from different massage tools. We also used menthol to replace the feeling of pain with tingling. In addition, we used other receptors, like smell and taste, to override the perception of the brain feeling pain.

Contrary to popular belief, your brain cannot multitask. If you give it two things to do, it has to give up one of them. In his case, we wanted it to give up pain, so we had to give it other things to do. After we find the right combination of receptors and senses to use, it just becomes about repetition. Just like learning a new skill, we had to get enough reps into the system for his brain to get good at something other than pain so it would become his default.

After a while, that is exactly what it did. After getting enough brain activation in his system, to give those other areas of the brain something else to do, his pain started to subside. The best part about it is that once he got out, he kept moving and experiencing the world around himself with those receptors and parts of the brain. That meant he naturally kept the pain away.

Once we get the ship righted and the brain back in order, it can take care of itself on its own as long as you keep the system tuned up. You can do so with regular movement like exercise, a good diet, and regular checkups to make sure your system is processing well.

This case highlights how important movement and brain activation can be to your life. It also allows us to understand how a lack of movement can change your brain and gives us a further understanding as to what someone with a lack of movement or feeling in a part of their body will need assistance with going forward. A lack of movement is not a death sentence, however, without movement a person will need to do things to supplement the activation the brain receives from movement to keep their brain and nervous system healthy.

The brain is an amazing piece of engineering; it will adapt and adjust to many difficulties. Even when things seem the most broken, there are options that can be chosen. It is important to keep those frontal lobes active so you can see these options when they come.

Our limbic brain is a common culprit—it is often taking resources away from our frontal lobes. In our office, we have a technique to deal with that part of the brain. NeuroEmotional Technique (NET) was developed by Dr. Scott Walker and works on the physiology of emotions and how they hijack the brain. This technique was developed to help the brain deal with past traumas, therefore making it so the limbic area does not require extra attention and resources. You see, the limbic brain can get stuck in traumas. With NET, we use a manual muscle test to see how your body is responding to the trauma. We pose certain test statements while testing the strength or coordination of a muscle. A strong or a weak muscle will indicate how the past trauma is affecting the way your body is working.

An example of NET might go like this: first we have the patient pose a statement like "I'm OK with healing." On the surface, most patients say something like "Of course I am OK with healing, that is why I am here." However, they are thinking that with their conscious brain. The muscle test looks closer at the unconscious or limbic brain.

We have the patient say the statement, "I'm OK with healing." If the muscle is strong, then they are congruent with that statement and we can move on. If the test shows the muscle going weak when they are saying that statement, this indicates that on some level they are not OK with it. With NET, we can then find out what might be causing them to be incongruent with the statement "I'm OK with healing."

Often times, in my experience, it comes back to a time they had to overcome something else hard—or, more often, a time when they failed to accomplish something hard. Their memory of that keeps playing in the background and can unconsciously affect the way they react to their world. It alters our emotional reality, which may or may not match up with actual reality. Our emotional reality is simply our emotional perception of the world around us. The energy of traumas that are stuck playing in the background affect our perception and ultimately how we react to the world.

When we have determined what trauma is affecting the body and how, we have the person focus their attention on the trauma while connecting to acupuncture meridian points. This technique is done without needles, simply by holding the acupuncture points with your fingers. This allows for the body to connect to those points and allow the energy to flow. This helps your brain make the connection that you are no longer going through this trauma anymore and allows the energy of that event to flow through the body and not get caught up or stuck in the tissues. Then the body can move past it. Once the brain can understand this, it is no longer triggered by that past event and no longer feels the need to devote resources toward staying safe from that past event, today. We can repeat this technique for multiple things that may be causing your body to hold onto past traumas.

All of these past traumas are replayed or stored in the limbic brain. That is the part of the brain that processes emotions and keeps us safe so we can make it to tomorrow. With the limbic system shut down, we are able to exercise the other parts of the brain, like the cerebellum and frontal lobe, to help move beyond trauma even more and to further get those areas of the brain to be more in the driver's seat. Remember, those areas are for emotional control and balance, and it is where happiness lives.

In one case in our office, we had a person who had been diagnosed with everything. She had been to about fifteen different doctors and each of them had given her a different diagnosis. She began to take them to heart and started to become those diagnoses.

She was no longer her given name. She was "Dysautonomia." She was "POTS." Her emotional reality had caused her to become the condition and no longer herself.

We had to do NET with her to remove the emotional charges around her getting those diagnoses. The diagnoses were tied to the way she felt when she had been bullied in school and called names. Remember that the limbic brain doesn't own a watch or a calendar. When the doctors began calling her "names" or giving her diagnoses, she felt helpless again like she did as a child and this caused her limbic brain and amygdala to hijack her thoughts and emotions. Once we were able to remove those triggers, we were able to work with making changes in her brain and move her past her traumas and help begin to heal.

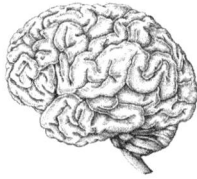

CHAPTER SIXTEEN

CLIENT SUCCESSES

In my career, I have been lucky to work with some pretty amazing people. Professional athletes are on another level—they have challenged me most and kept me sharp. Even when rehabbing from an injury, their brains and movements are on another level. I would frequently find myself having to reinvent therapies. Some of the things they would make look easy were impossible for most patients. If you want to challenge yourself and your thought process, that is a great demographic to practice with. They will keep you on your toes.

Kids make my job fun and rewarding, and they pick up the whole office. When they win in their treatment, everyone gets excited. They have that innocence about them that helps them overcome their obstacles, which is really cool to see. And some of them you watch grow up right before your eyes. Their pain and struggle make them stronger, and often puts them ahead of their peers in maturity. Plus, they are a blank slate and don't come in with any preconceived notions about whether this will work or not. They come in and do the work and get better.

Kids' brains are sponges for things like applied clinical neuroscience. Their brains learn new tasks so quickly you can really work through a lot of things in a hurry. It is amazing, sometimes, to see how fast their brain changes with some really complex tasks. You can take a kid who cannot read because his eyes will not move in sync and have him reading the whole Harry Potter series in a couple weeks. With adults, those same changes might take a couple months because sometimes it is harder to unlearn something the body has done improperly for years than it is to teach it the right way the first time. Kids really are a treat to work with for that reason.

I couldn't fly in the Navy, but I still got the opportunity to be a part of that world in some way when I had the opportunity to work with some elite soldiers from the Navy SEALs. Our veterans have a really special place in my heart, I think because that avenue was ripped out from under me. Their spirit and intensity always amaze me.

One soldier that I have worked with recently is Matt, a Navy SEAL Medic. It was his job to respond to emergencies on the base. He suffered a diffuse axonal injury in a car accident responding to a call on base, the most severe brain injury that you can have. When he emerged from his coma, he was severely limited in his function. He was confined to a wheelchair, unable to speak—but he wanted to heal, and he put in the work.

He pushed himself harder than any of his doctors. He has had some truly amazing neuro doctors, speech therapists, physical therapists, etc., and he grew in leaps and bounds. My wife, also a chiropractor specializing in NET, and I were brought in to work with him because they felt there was something emotionally holding him back. Aside from the accident and trauma of being a Navy SEAL, he also had some previous traumas in his life as a child and he seemed to be stuck on them. We were brought in to use NET and functional neurology to remove some of those triggers, to shut down that limbic response, and to allow his cognitive brain to flourish.

And it did. Once he stopped worrying so much about his past trauma, his cognition kicked into another gear. Thankfully, he has an amazing wife who left no stone unturned when it came to working to help her husband. She was the one who realized he seemed to be stuck in the past and advocated to get his care moving in that direction. She knew that even though he was getting better, there was more inside of him that needed to get dealt with. He is still healing and on his journey, but the NET and removing emotions has allowed him to be able to move better and take his treatments to another level. He has been able to walk and, with some assistance, was even able to cut the grass, which was something he really wanted to do.

I have chosen a few more stories to help outline how amazing the brain is and how it can make some pretty incredible changes. These case studies will help showcase some of the important concepts we have talked about in the "science" sections in pretty intense detail. The saying goes, "A picture tells a thousand words." Well, I hope these case studies help paint a picture of the amazing abilities of your brain.

These are the stories of people who came to us as a last resort. These are stories of people who were told to accept their new normal but refused to accept the limitations that were put upon them, and as a result were able to improve their quality of life and take back control of their health.

The Limbic Brain

The limbic brain can really take over and control us. One patient, an active and successful young woman who enjoyed playing soccer, came to us presenting with a complaint of violent head-shakes. Her head would shake involuntarily in response to loud sounds, objects flying at her in the air or on the ground, and especially finger snapping. Yep, the sound of snapping fingers would elicit violent "headshakes," as she referred to them. And they *were* violent. She would shake her head like a punk rocker head banging—but side to side. This uncontrollable reaction was negatively affecting her job and her soccer hobby, to the point where both were becoming impossible.

We discovered this reaction was tied to the fact that she had recently been in a horrible car accident while driving across a bridge. The last thing she remembered before the crash was see-ing the other driver's face as they collided and both went careen-ing off the side of the road. The next thing she knew, paramedics were snapping their fingers to bring her back. Her car was laying on its side, off the road. They took her to the hospital to check her out for concussion and other injuries. When she arrived, a police officer had come up to ask her some questions about the accident. Being the kindhearted person that she was, she asked the officer about the other driver. She wanted to know if he was alright.

The officer replied, "No, he did not make it, but that is how he wanted it." She looked at him, puzzled. The officer contin-ued, "We found a note in his car. A suicide note. He was on that road to take his own life. He chose your car to kill himself with."

Think about the emotional and physiological implications that would have on your mental health and well-being. Not only to know that someone died in a car accident with you, but that they *used* you to purposefully kill themselves.

Her limbic brain had stored that memory alongside the movement. In the car accident, she rolled her car, and in a rollover your head is violently whipped from side to side. Remember that thoughts and emotions travel through and are regulated by the same parts of our brains as our movements are. Her violent headshakes back and forth were very similar to the violent shaking her head and neck went through in the car accident.

Together, we came to the conclusion that her movements in response to loud stimuli and snapping fingers was a regression back to that time. Remember that the limbic brain doesn't own a watch. It can't tell time, and it also doesn't know dates. It only knows survival, and only realizes right now. So, with those noises, her limbic brain was back in the car with the same emotional reality, but also the same movement patterns. We have to break that limbic cycle and properly process those emotions, and *then* we can go in and properly work through the movement patterns as well.

In her case, we used NeuroEmotional Technique. In this patient's case, she was stuck in the emotional reality that she was not safe. Every stimulus in the environment kept driving that fear mindset into her more and more. Every object that came near her was threatening, and every finger snap took her back to the moment after the car accident. These triggers made her relive the trauma and all the emotion that went along with it. We did a lot of NET and repatterned her brain, changing her physiological reactions to those stimuli. When we released the hold that the trauma had on her, we could quiet the limbic system.

Another question we often get is, "How do you turn on the frontal lobe or the cerebellum?" The short answer is to do things that use that part of the brain. So, since we know the frontal lobe does movement, do movement. The longer answer is that each movement can affect that part of the brain differently. That is where the years of study and paying attention to detail come in. The trick is finding specifically what movements, at what frequency, what amplitude, what wavelength, and at what depth would work. For this patient, it was all about doing movements with her eyes in very small increments, and very slowly at first, to get her brain to feel comfortable and able to respond to the environment from a place of safety instead of fear. We started by playing catch, and then by having her follow targets around a room, and then we were able to have objects and targets move right at her. At every step, her care was specifically tailored to what her brain could handle at the time.

After two weeks doing the work and removing her triggers, she was able to kick around the soccer ball with her friends. Very quickly, she went from violently shaking her head at anything that came at her to voluntarily playing soccer without a headshake in sight. Her tears of joy streamed as she told me how she overcame this struggle and discovered another layer of strength to herself.

Jay and Greg: Epigenetics

As we discussed in the section on epigenetics, our genes do not get the final say in how our cells express themselves. One of our patients showed genetic markers for Parkinson's disease in a blood test. In addition, his brother also showed signs of the condition. He was determined to beat the condition and came to us having already put together a pretty good plan of how he was going to beat it. He had looked into many different types of therapies and had even purchased some at-home tools, like a vibration plate.

Unlike many people, Jay did not accept the sentence of Parkinson's disease, even with the genetic markers. He worked hard and, using the principles of applied clinical neuroscience, we were able to overcome his genes by changing the early immediate gene response. We used chiropractic adjustments and specific neurological therapies to rewrite his story and rewire his brain. After just a couple weeks, his tremors stopped while standing. Then his tremors went away while laying down, and he started to get better sleep. By the time he left us after two weeks, you would not know he had Parkinson's disease if you looked at him.

Jay kept in touch for quite a while. His symptoms stayed away, and he was able to return to the active lifestyle he enjoyed before his diagnosis.

Another patient, Greg, had a different genetic anomaly: a condition called hereditary spastic paraplegia that would eventually cause him to lose the use of his legs. When he first came to us, he had already progressed years into his condition: his legs were already very tight and painful. His goals when we started with care were just to have a little better balance so he could dress himself. He didn't want to be such a burden on his lovely wife.

He showed genetic markers for this condition, yet during his treatment of just one week, he was able to feel his feet for the first time in twelve years. That was on Wednesday. On Friday, he danced with his wife for the first time in fifteen years in our back office. Everyone was crying. His new goal upon leaving our office was to get back on the ice to skate with his grandkids.

Before long, he was skating.

In both of these cases, if genes were the whole story then treatment would have been pointless. But that was not the case for either of these men. They believed there were other options out there for them, did their research, put in the work, and surpassed all the expectations that were put upon them. With both of them, we used treatments that activated the receptors in their bodies to affect neuroplastic change in their brains. That is, we turned up the sensory stimuli or way they were feeling, hearing, and seeing the world.

To accomplish this, we put both of them on a vibration platform to activate the muscles much more. We were then able to have them move on a beat, like dancing. Dancing makes you use your eyes, ears, muscles, and joints to feel, see, and hear your environment as you move around it. Practicing doing so helps give your brain even more information to make your response more appropriate and easier. For both of them, this was a huge change in the way their bodies and brains felt about their surroundings and how they moved around it. It changed the job of the cell and forced them to make different proteins to meet the new requirements, altering the way their DNA was expressed.

Remember: a doctor's opinion is just that, an opinion. That is why we can get a second opinion or a third. If a doctor doesn't give you the answer you resonate with, we don't have to take it as law.

Neuroplastic Change Case Study: Ryan and Brain Maps

Concussions have been a hot topic in recent years and have been the focus of a lot of research in neuroscience. Since the discovery of chronic traumatic encephalopathy (CTE), many have raced to get a better understanding of what happens to the brain during concussions. Some of the hallmark signs and symptoms of concussion, like headache, dizziness, and cognitive difficulties, may not be the only signs that the brain is damaged or struggling to recover from injury. Plus, the fact that each successive concussion is usually worse (meaning that they seem to have an additive effect) would lead one to believe that maybe the brain does not "heal" from concussions but simply finds

NEVER ACCEPT YOUR NEW NORMAL

a way to adapt with having one. It essentially rewires itself to maintain function. This sheds some light on the amazing ability of the brain to maintain the status quo, even when faced with something that damages it so profoundly. Even with damage to tissue that is vital to some brain function, the brain is able to rewire itself to keep you living and doing what you need to do.

One way that we measure brain function currently is to perform a quantitative Electroencephalogram (EEG). This is that test where you put on what looks like a swimming cap with a bunch of wires attached. The cap and its machine measure brain waves.

You will remember back in the chapter on frequency that brain waves are the way your cells communicate with each other. The EEG allows us to measure those brain waves and determine whether or not they are in healthy patterns.

That brings us to another patient experience. Ryan was sixteen when he had come to us. He got a concussion while playing soccer and, like most sixteen-year-olds, didn't think anything of it. Just like I did after my big injury, Ryan actually continued playing that game. After the game, he was complaining about a bad headache and a little dizziness, so his parents took him to the hospital where they did a CT scan. The doctors ruled out a brain bleed or anything more serious and diagnosed him with a mild concussion. At that time, the normal treatment for concussion was to sit in a dark room with no stimuli. FYI, that is not the currently accepted standard of care (and really wasn't at the time, either, but that is for another book).

Anyway, after a few weeks, the easy-to-tell symptoms like headache and dizziness wore off. He cleared the return-to-play protocols but was still having issues. His grades were suffering, and his mood had changed significantly. His mother, friends, and family members reported these changes, but Ryan didn't really notice them as much—then again, in my experience I have not met many sixteen-year-old boys who are very in touch with their feelings.

Another way to look at brain waves is like this. In an unhealthy person the EEG might be chaotic. The information or frequency being passed from cell to cell in the brain might be random and incoherent. However, in a healthier person you will see coherence of the brain waves and information being passed. This means that the brain waves and the function of the brain are synchronized.

The best symphony orchestra is always playing together at the same time, to the same beat, and on the same page. A bad orchestra would be out of sync and would sound like a mess. Well, in an unhealthy brain, the signals that are being sent are out of time and out of sync with everything else, and the result is much more "mess" than it is "symphony."

In this case, the young man originally showed brain waves that were consistent with that of a child with ADHD. Following treatment of just two weeks, he showed brain wave patterns that were more consistent with a healthy, in sync, "symphonic" brain. Now, we have always known that this sort of change is possible with neurofeedback and intense therapy, but with conventional measures it can take up to twelve weeks to see changes like that.

We did it in two. Here's how:

We did a lot of work on his cerebellum. That is the conductor of the brain's orchestra. Your cerebellum is responsible for keeping everything in line, on time, and functioning beautifully. With a good cerebellum, the music sounds more like Mozart, but when the cerebellum breaks down it can sound a lot more like "Symphony of Destruction."

When working with the cerebellum, you need to challenge the movement and balance centers together. With Ryan, we used a giant spinning chair called the GyroStim. The GyroStim allows us to move a client through space to activate receptors in a very specific way. Depending on which direction we spin the person, we can be very specific about which parts of the brain we are turning on. This kind of therapy is much more specific than medication. It can be very difficult to know exactly what areas of the brain will be affected by medications—which is why side effects are so common. With this therapy, and the other therapies we use, we can be very specific about what is getting turned on or off.

With the cerebellum being all about balance, coordination, and speed, using things like the GyroStim can allow us to specifically affect the cerebellum. This also allows us to turn up the depth and amplitude of the client's treatment to match what he can handle. While he was spinning, he had to shoot targets that were outside of the machine with a laser. This forced not only his cerebellum to coordinate this movement between his eyes and hand, but also it involved the frontal lobe to initiate the movement, other parts of his brain and body. This all helped his brain understand how he was moving through space. For him, we wanted to incorporate a lot of stimuli and activities to activate the most brain we could. His system needed that bigger amplitude and more depth to get the brain to "wake up" and do its jobs better and more efficiently. This improved brain function and efficiency led him all the way to realizing his goals. He ended up as the kicker at a university and played football at a really high level. He flourished both on the field and in the classroom.

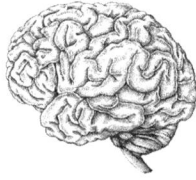

CHAPTER SEVENTEEN

THE END

In health care, people and patients come to us for answers. It can sometimes be a pretty heavy responsibility when someone sits in front of you, broken and scared, looking for answers—and more importantly, looking for hope. Hope is a very powerful tool, and it can be wielded for good or for bad, even with the best intentions.

When this weight gets too heavy, I have to think back to something I learned in school: the meaning of the word "doctor." The word comes from the Latin *docere,* meaning, "to teach." Guide us toward knowledge, but in the end doesn't necessarily teach us facts but instead how to learn and how to find facts. In the same way, that is the job of the doctor: to be a guide in your journey to health. A doctor's job is not to always have the last answer but instead to be a soundboard and director of your questions and your search for knowledge on health and well-being.

This is maybe a different model than what a lot of us believe in, but this *has* to be the relationship between doctor and patient going forward. This is how we get to the world where "diagnosis" is more of a verb than a noun. We can offer answers when possible, but for true health it is really up to the patient to continue their quest for more answers and more knowledge. It is up to the patient to take ownership for their health.

Above all, the doctor should offer hope and, even if they do not have the answer, a means to seek out the person or resource who might. I do not always have the answers for patients (and another of my biggest flaws might be in not always admitting that), but it doesn't mean that an answer is not out there. The landscape of health care changes daily, our understanding of the body and brain are always changing and evolving, and we need to constantly stay on top of the most current information, understanding that even that might be obsolete the next day.

There is always hope that there is something else around the corner. There is always hope that our understanding might shift and allow for new possibilities, even if it is beyond our understanding. We just need to connect with someone who can help us understand.

Connection is, after all, what health is really all about. Connecting our neurological pathways, connecting to our meaning, connecting to our purpose, connecting to others, and connecting to our future. This will help us make stronger connections in our brain.

So, in a way, when we are "reconnecting" pathways in the brain with the work that we do in our office, we are talking about so much more. Reconnecting to society. Reconnecting to your purpose. Reconnecting to the earth and nature. Reconnecting to healthy food. Reconnecting to healthy relationships, reconnecting to play, and ultimately reconnecting to hope and love. All of these reconnections will reconnect you to yourself, and to your health.

The bottom line, in all these lessons and case stories, is that you can Never Accept Your New Normal.

The information will change, and we will evolve, but if our thought process is sound and we continue to question and move forward, our technique will evolve with it. Patients will keep you on the cutting edge, learning more and more every day. It can be very easy to get caught up in some of the academics and research, but if your focus is on the people, then you will always be learning and striving to do better. So, even if some of the information in this book is obsolete by the time you read it, I hope you are still left with a will to fight, advocate, move forward, and question everything. That will never be obsolete.

A lot of times, we drive so hard and with such intention but don't listen to ourselves to make sure we are still going the right direction. Progress for the sake of progress is not always what is best for the soul. Drive is necessary, but also not the only thing. Such is our duality; we have a left and right brain. One side is the drive and intention, that is the left. The other side is the fun, big-picture brain that is the right. They both need to be fed and both need to be given the spotlight at different times. Stopping and listening once in a while is the only way to really know which path to take. It is really easy to put your head down and push through. It can be harder to stop and smell the roses, to wait and make sure you are still headed in the direction that brings joy to your life.

Ultimately, struggle is a part of all our lives, but it is a necessary part that forces us to grow and evolve and become something greater than what we were the day before. The challenges we face can define us, not by what they have done *to* us but by what they have done *for* us. In the end, we are a collection of the memories that we have made and the mountains that we have climbed. Our experiences are so much a part of who we are that they determine how we see the world. If we look at the challenges and struggles of life with a negative lens, we end up getting beaten down by them and it can feel as though life is happening to us and against us. If we choose to find the meaning in the struggles and rise above them, to look at them as things that are done for us as opportunities to grow and evolve, we can see things in a better, more positive light.

The brain will do what you tell it to—even more, it will get really good at what you tell it to. So, we can build those pathways around movement of the body, mind, and spirit into evolution for the good, or we can build those pathways around staying scared and fearful, never getting outside our comfort zone. Sometimes we need to dance within the flames and experience what it feels like to get burned so we can experience life to its fullest. Giving up, accepting a new normal, and not taking chances is safe, but does not allow for growth and evolution.

Keep pushing, exercise your brain every day, and Never Accept Your New Normal!

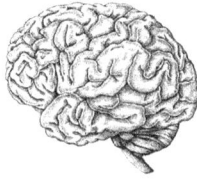

WORKS CITED PAGE

Amplitude: Definition of Amplitude by Oxford Dictionary on Lexico.com also meaning of Amplitude. (n.d.). Retrieved from https://en.oxforddictionaries.com/definition/Amplitude

Arnett DK, Blumenthal RS, Albert MA, et al. 2019 ACC/AHA Guideline on the Primary Prevention of Cardiovascular Disease: A Report of the American College of Cardiology/American Heart Association Task Force on Clinical Practice Guidelines [published correction appears in Circulation. 2019 Sep 10;140(11):e649-e650] [published correction appears in Circulation. 2020 Jan 28;141(4):e60] [published correction appears in Circulation. 2020 Apr 21;141(16):e774]. Circulation. 2019;140(11):e596-e646. DOI:10.1161/CIR.0000000000000678

Benjamin EJ, Muntner P, Alonso A, Bittencourt MS, Callaway CW, Carson AP, et al. Heart disease and stroke statistics—2019 update: a report from the American Heart Association. Circulation. 2019;139(10):e56–528

Bitsko, R. H., Holbrook, J. R., Ghandour, R. M., Blumberg, S. J., Visser, S. N., Perou, R., & Walkup, J. T. (2018). Epidemiology and Impact of Health Care Provider–Diagnosed Anxiety and Depression Among US Children. *Journal of Developmental & Behavioral Pediatrics, 39*(5), 395-403. doi:10.1097/dbp.0000000000000571

Standing outside the fire [CD]. (n.d.).

Cree RA, Bitsko RH, Robinson LR, Holbrook JR, Danielson ML, Smith DS, Kaminski JW, Kenney MK, Peacock G. Health care, family, and community factors associated with mental, behavioral, and developmental disorders and poverty among children aged 2–8 years—the United States, 2016. MMWR, 2018;67(5):1377-1383.

Danielson, M. L., Bitsko, R. H., Ghandour, R. M., Holbrook, J. R., Kogan, M. D., & Blumberg, S. J. (2018). Prevalence of Parent-Reported ADHD Diagnosis and Associated Treatment Among U.S. Children and Adolescents, 2016. *Journal of Clinical Child & Adolescent Psychology, 47*(2), 199-212. doi:10.1080/15374416.2017.1417860

Data and Statistics on Children's Mental Health. (2020, June 15). Retrieved from https://www.cdc.gov/childrensmentalhealth/data.html

Depression. (n.d.). Retrieved from https://www.nimh.nih.gov/health/topics/depression/index.shtml

Depth: Definition of Depth by Oxford Dictionary on Lexico. com also meaning of Depth. (n.d.). Retrieved from https:// en.oxforddictionaries.com/definition/depth

Dracobly, A. (2004). Review: A Cultural History of Medical Vitalism in Enlightenment Montpellier. *Journal of the History of Medicine and Allied Sciences, 59*(1), 149-150. doi:10.1093/jhmas/jrg045

Frankl, V. E., Lasch, I., Kushner, H. S., & Winslade, W. J. (2019). *Mans search for meaning*. Boston: Beacon Press.

Frequency: Definition of Frequency by Oxford Dictionary on Lexico.com also meaning of Frequency. (n.d.). Retrieved from https://en.oxforddictionaries.com/definition/frequency

Fryar CD, Chen T-C, Li X. Prevalence of uncontrolled risk factors for cardiovascular disease: the United States, 1999–2010 pdf icon[PDF-494K]. NCHS data brief, no. 103. Hyattsville, MD: National Center for Health Statistics; 2012. Accessed May 9, 2019.

Gesundheit! (n.d.). Retrieved from https://www.patchadams. org/gesundheit/

Ghandour, R. M., Sherman, L. J., Vladutiu, C. J., Ali, M. M., Lynch, S. E., Bitsko, R. H., & Blumberg, S. J. (2019). Prevalence and Treatment of Depression, Anxiety, and Conduct Problems in US Children. *The Journal of Pediatrics, 206*. doi:10.1016/j.jpeds.2018.09.021

Heart Disease Facts. (2020, September 08). Retrieved from https://www.cdc.gov/heartdisease/facts.htm

Heron, M. Deaths: Leading causes for 2017 pdf icon[PDF – 3 M]. National Vital Statistics Reports;68(6). Accessed November 19, 2019.

Horowitz, A. M., Fan, X., Bieri, G., Smith, L. K., Sanchez-Diaz, C. I., Schroer, A. B.,...Villeda, S. A. (2020). Blood factors transfer beneficial effects of exercise on neurogenesis and cognition to the aged brain. *Science, 369*(6500), 167-173. doi:10.1126/science.aaw2622

Ignácio, Z. M., Silva, R. S., Plissari, M. E., Quevedo, J., & Réus, G. Z. (2019). Physical Exercise and Neuroinflammation in Major Depressive Disorder. *Molecular Neurobiology, 56*(12), 8323-8335. doi:10.1007/s12035-019-01670-1

Ioannidis, J. P. (2008). Effectiveness of antidepressants: An evidence myth constructed from a thousand randomized trials? *Philosophy, Ethics, and Humanities in Medicine, 3*(1), 14. doi:10.1186/1747-5341-3-14

Key Substance Use and Mental Health Indicators in the... (n.d.). Retrieved from https://www.samhsa.gov/data/sites/default/files/cbhsq-reports/NSDUHNational FindingsReport2018/NSDUHNationalFindingsReport 2018.pdf

Kochanek KD, Murphy SL, Xu JQ, Arias E. Deaths: Final data for 2017. National Vital

Statistics Reports; vol 68 no 9. Hyattsville, MD: National Center for Health Statistics. 2019.

Pascoe, M., Bailey, A. P., Craike, M., Carter, T., Patten, R., Stepto, N., & Parker, A. (2020). Physical activity and exercise in youth mental health promotion: A scoping review. *BMJ Open Sport & Exercise Medicine, 6*(1). doi:10.1136/bmjsem-2019-000677

Perez, E. C., Bravo, D. R., Rodgers, S. P., Khan, A. R., & Leasure, J. L. (2019). Shaping the adult brain with exercise during development: Emerging evidence and knowledge gaps. *International Journal of Developmental Neuroscience, 78*(1), 147-155. doi:10.1016/j.ijdevneu.2019.06.006

Perou R, Bitsko RH, Blumberg SJ, Pastor P, Ghandour RM, Gfroerer JC, Hedden SL, Crosby AE, Visser SN, Schieve LA, Parks SE, Hall JE, Brody D, Simile CM, Thompson WW, Baio J, Avenevoli S, Kogan MD, Huang LN. Mental health surveillance among children—the United States, 2005—2011. MMWR 2013;62(Suppl; May 16, 2013):1-35.

Rocke, A. J. (2020, July 27). Friedrich Wöhler. Retrieved from https://www.britannica.com/biography/Friedrich-Wohler

Sharma, B., Allison, D., Tucker, P., Mabbott, D., & Timmons, B. W. (2019). Cognitive and neural effects of exercise following traumatic brain injury: A systematic review of randomized and controlled clinical trials. *Brain Injury, 34*(2), 149-159. doi:10.1080/02699052.2019.1683892

Siegel, R. L., Miller, K. D., & Jemal, A. (2018). Cancer statistics, 2018. *CA: A Cancer Journal for Clinicians, 68*(1), 7-30. doi:10.3322/caac.21442

Substance Abuse and Mental Health Services Administration. Key substance use and mental health

indicators in the United States: Results from the 2018 National Survey on Drug Use and Health

(HHS Publication No. PEP19-5068, NSDUH Series H-54). Rockville, MD: Center for Behavioral Health Statistics and Quality, Retrieved from https://www.samhsa.gov/data/ (2019)

Tone: Definition of Tone by Oxford Dictionary on Lexico. com also meaning of Tone. (n.d.). Retrieved from https:// en.oxforddictionaries.com/definition/Tone

Visser, S. N., Danielson, M. L., Bitsko, R. H., Perou, R., & Blumberg, S. J. (2013). Convergent Validity of Parent-Reported Attention-Deficit/Hyperactivity Disorder Diagnosis. *JAMA Pediatrics, 167*(7), 674. doi:10.1001/ jamapediatrics.2013.2364

Vitalism. (n.d.). Retrieved from https://www.merriam-webster. com/dictionary/vitalism.

Wavelength: Definition of Wavelength by Oxford Dictionary on Lexico.com also meaning of Wavelength. (n.d.). Retrieved from https://en.oxforddictionaries.com/definition/wavelength

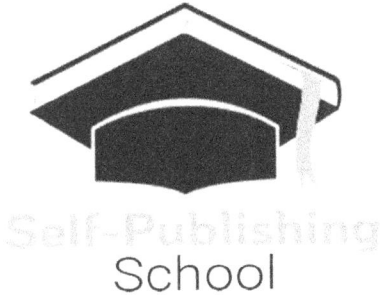

Self-Publishing

School

NOW IT'S YOUR TURN

Discover the EXACT 3-step blueprint you need to become a bestselling author in as little as 3 months.

Self-Publishing School helped me, and now I want them to help you with this FREE resource to begin outlining your book!

Even if you're busy, bad at writing, or don't know where to start, you CAN write a bestseller and build your best life.

With tools and experience across a variety of niches and professions, Self-Publishing School is the only resource you need to take your book to the finish line!

DON'T WAIT

Say "YES" to becoming a bestseller:

https://self-publishingschool.com/friend/

Follow the steps on the page to get a FREE resource to get started on your book and unlock a discount to get started with Self-Publishing School

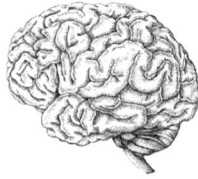

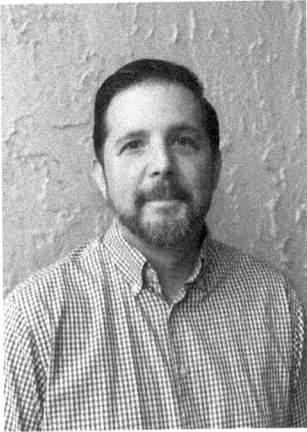

Dr. Longyear has dedicated his life to studying the brain and nervous system and how it impacts our health and happiness. He is the director of Applied Clinical Neuroscience at the NeuroLIFE Institute with Life University in Marietta, GA as well as Brain Optimization Institute in Jacksonville, Florida. In the clinical setting he works with complex neurological conditions using Chiropractic, Applied Clinical Neuroscience, and Functional Medicine to give hope to some of the most difficult cases that have been told to accept their new normal. In addition to working with patients, he also works with the research department at Life University to examine and develop new and innovative ways to use the principles of neuroplasticity to restore health and function to the brain and nervous system for patients with a wide variety of conditions. He also has developed curriculum for Applied Clinical Neuroscience and teaches a certificate program at the school and travels all over the world teaching doctors how to use these techniques with BrainDC.

When he is not working with Functional Neurology, he spends time with his wife and two dogs roaming the beach as well as relaxing in the sand. You might find him on the beach with kite and board hitting some waves.

Can You Help?

Thank You for Reading My Book!

I really appreciate all of your feedback, and
I love hearing what you have to say.

I need your input to make the next version of
this book and my future books better.

Please leave me an honest review on Amazon
letting me know what you thought of the book.

Thanks so much!

Dr. Michael Longyear